I0350842

Deleuze, Guattari and the Schizoanalysis of the Global Pandemic

Schizoanalytic Applications

Series Editors: Ian Buchanan, Marcelo Svirsky and David Savat

Schizoanalysis has the potential to be to Deleuze and Guattari's work what deconstruction is to Derrida's – the standard rubric by which their work is known and, more importantly, applied. Many within the field of Deleuze and Guattari studies would resist this idea, but the goal of this series is to broaden the base of scholars interested in their work. Deleuze and Guattari's ideas are widely known and used, but not in a systematic way and this is both a strength and weakness. It is a strength because it enables people to pick up their work from a wide variety of perspectives, but it is also a weakness because it makes it difficult to say with any clarity what exactly a 'Deleuzo–Guattarian' approach is. This has inhibited the uptake of Deleuze and Guattari's thinking in the more wilful disciplines such as history, politics and even philosophy. Without this methodological core, Deleuze and Guattari studies risk becoming simply another intellectual fashion that will soon be superseded by newer figures.

The goal of the Schizoanalytic Applications series is to create a methodological core and build a sustainable model of schizoanalysis that will attract new scholars to the field. With this purpose, the series also aims to be at the forefront of the field by starting a discussion about the nature of Deleuze and Guattari's methodology.

Titles published in the series:

Deleuze and the Schizoanalysis of Feminism, edited by Janae Sholtz and Cheri Carr

Deleuze and the Schizoanalysis of Literature, edited by Ian Buchanan, Tim Matts and Aidan Tynan

Deleuze and the Schizoanalysis of Religion, edited by Lindsay Powell-Jones and F. LeRon Shults

Deleuze and the Schizoanalysis of Visual Art, edited by Ian Buchanan and Lorna Collins

Deleuze, Guattari and the Schizoanalysis of Trans Studies, edited by Ciara Cremin

Deleuze, Guattari and the Schizoanalysis of Postmedia, edited by Joff P. N. Bradley, Alex Taek-Gwang Lee and Manoj N. Y.

Deleuze, Guattari and the Schizoanalysis of the Global Pandemic

Revolutionary Praxis and Neoliberal Crisis

Edited by

Saswat Samay Das and Ananya Roy Pratihar

BLOOMSBURY ACADEMIC
LONDON • NEW YORK • OXFORD • NEW DELHI • SYDNEY

BLOOMSBURY ACADEMIC
Bloomsbury Publishing Plc
50 Bedford Square, London, WC1B 3DP, UK
1385 Broadway, New York, NY 10018, USA
29 Earlsfort Terrace, Dublin 2, Ireland

BLOOMSBURY, BLOOMSBURY ACADEMIC and the Diana logo are trademarks of Bloomsbury Publishing Plc

First published in Great Britain 2023
This paperback edition published 2024

Cover design by Charlotte Daniels
Cover image: Abstract landscape background
(© StudioM1 / iStock / Getty Images Plus);
Dance Kathexis (© Stelios Bakhlavas)

A catalogue record for this book is available from the British Library.

A catalog record for this book is available from the Library of Congress.

Library of Congress Control Number: 2023937742.

ISBN: HB: 978-1-3502-7691-8
PB: 978-1-3502-7739-7
ePDF: 978-1-3502-7740-3
eBook: 978-1-3502-7741-0

Series: Schizoanalytic Applications

Typeset by RefineCatch Limited, Bungay, Suffolk

Contents

Figures

Contributors

Brent Adkins is Professor of Philosophy at Roanoke College in Salem, Virginia, USA. His primary interests are nineteenth- and twentieth-century European philosophy, Modern Philosophy and politics. His books include *Death and Desire in Hegel, Heidegger and Deleuze* (2007), *True Freedom: Spinoza's Practical Philosophy* (2009) and, with Paul Hinlicky, *Rethinking Philosophy & Theology with Deleuze: A New Cartography* (2013). He recently published Deleuze and Guattari's *A Thousand Plateaus: A Reader's Guide and Critical Introduction* (2015) and *A Guide to Ethics and Moral Philosophy* (2017).

Francisco J. Alcalá is a postdoctoral researcher of the Margarita Salas programme at the University of Barcelona, in the Philosophy Department (Aporía group). His research interests focus on contemporary French philosophy, particularly on Gilles Deleuze, the author around whom he has articulated the different lines of his research, demonstrating a particular interest in the intersection of the strictly theoretical or metaphysical side and the socio-political and cultural side of philosophical thought.

Clayton Crockett is professor in the Department of Philosophy and Religion and the Director of the interdisciplinary Religious Studies program. He regularly teaches courses on Exploring Religion; Philosophy of Religion; Religion, Science and Technology; and Religion and Psychology. He has authored or edited a number of books, including *Religion, Politics and the Earth* (2012); *The Future of Continental Philosophy of Religion* (2014) and, most recently, *Derrida After the End of Writing* (2017).

Brad Evans is a political philosopher, critical theorist, and writer, who specializes on the problem of violence. He is author of over 20 books and edited volumes, including most recently *Ecce Humanitas: Beholding the Pain of Humanity* (Columbia University Press, 2020). He previously led a dedicated columns/series on violence in both the New York Times and the Los Angeles Review of Books. Brad currently serves as Chair of Political Violence and Aesthetics at the University of Bath, United Kingdom, where is he founder and director of the Centre for the Study of Violence. He is also the co-host of Books with BraNd, a live and recorded show with the comedian and actor Russell Brand where they explore timeless literary classics.

Emine Görgül is an associate professor and former vice-chair in Istanbul Technical University-ITU Department of Interior Architecture. She has been the chair of 'Deleuze Studies Conference Istanbul 2014', and also a keynote presenter and camp tutor at many Deleuze Studies conferences. She has authored numerous articles and book chapters, both in Turkish and in English, on design education and innovative interventions, architecture theory and criticism, gender and space, design culture and urban interiors. She has been nominated and included in *Who's Who in the World Index* for the 2016 volume.

Jernej Markelj is a lecturer in New Media and Digital Culture at the University of Amsterdam. In 2020, he defended his PhD thesis, which offered a reevaluation of Gilles Deleuze's immanent ethics from the perspective of illusions of consciousness. Jernej's work has been published in edited books such as *Clickbait Capitalism: Economies of Desire in the Twenty-First Century* and in academic journals including *New Media & Society*, *Convergence* and *The Journal of Media Art Study and Theory*.

Chantal Meza is an abstract painter living and working in the United Kingdom. Her work has featured in Exhibitions, Auctions, Interventions, Biennale & Donations in prominent Museums and Galleries in Mexico, Paraguay and the United Kingdom. Her work is held in private and public collections. She has delivered International Lectures & Seminars at reputable Universities and been commissioned publicly and privately. Her artwork features in many prominent international outlets as well as on book covers, digital and print magazines. Her current projects include the State of Disappearance art book to be published in 2023 and the commissioned feature artist of 'Books with BraNd' – a live and recorded show with Russell Brand and Brad Evans.

Kyle J. Novak is Postdoctoral Research Fellow with the 'Deleuze and Cosmology Research Group' at Laurentian University in Sudbury, Ontario. He is also an instructor at the University of Guelph, where he attained his doctorate degree in Philosophy in 2021 with a dissertation on *Gilles Deleuze's Non-ontological Philosophy*. His publications on Deleuze have appeared in *The Journal of Speculative Philosophy*, *Symposium: The Canadian Journal of Continental Philosophy*, *Philosophy Today*, and in the volume *Werner Herzog and Philosophy* (2020).

Paul Patton is Hongyi Chair Professor of Philosophy in School of Philosophy at Wuhan University. He has authored *Deleuze and the Political* (2000) and *Deleuzian Concepts: Philosophy, Colonization, Politics* (2010). He is a Fellow of the Australian Academy of the Humanities and is currently Editor of the *Journal of Social and Political Philosophy*. He edited *Deleuze: A Critical Reader* (Blackwell 1996) and co-edited *Between Deleuze and Derrida*, (Continuum, 2003), *Deleuze and the Postcolonial* (Edinburgh 2010) and *Deleuze and Pragmatism*, (Routledge 2015).

Patricia Pisters is Professor of Film Studies and Media Culture at the University of Amsterdam. She is one of the founding editors of the peer-reviewed *Open Access Journal NECSUS: European Journal of Media Studies*. With Bernd Herzogenrath, she is series editor of *Thinking I Media* at Bloomsbury; with Wanda Strauven and Malte Hagener, series editor of *Film Culture in Transition*. Her most recent book is *New Blood in Contemporary Cinema: Women Directors and the Poetics of Horror* (2022).

Virgilio A. Rivas holds a PhD on F. W. J. Schelling and the broader relation of German Idealism to the current Anthropocene debate and extinction and collapse theory. His research interests intersect with Deleuze Studies, critical theory, posthumanism, environmental humanities, island studies and research into indigenous cultures. He teaches philosophy at the Polytechnic University of the Philippines.

Ananya Roy Pratihar is an Assistant Professor in Communication Studies at the Institute of Management and Information Science, Bhubaneswar, India. She has jointly edited *Technology, Urban Space and Network Community* (2022). She is currently editing a special Issue for *Deleuze and Guattari Studies* and an edited collection *Deleuze, Guattari and the Schizoanalysis of Post-Neoliberalism* (2023). Her research interests include Decolonial Studies, Deleuze Studies, Film Studies, Eco-humanism and Cultural Studies.

Saswat Samay Das is an Associate Professor in the Department of Humanities and Social Sciences, Indian Institute of Technology, Kharagpur, India. His research interest areas are Postcolonial and Postmodern Studies, Continental Thinking, Deleuze Studies, Political Activism, Social Movement, Critical Theory and Radical Neo-Marxism. He has jointly authored *Taking Place of Language* (2013) and has jointly edited *Technology, Urban Space and the Networked Community, Deleuze and the Global Terror* (2022). He is currently editing a Special Issue for *Deleuze and Guattari Studies* and an edited book *Deleuze, Guattari and the Schizoanalysis of Post-Neoliberalism*. He has published in well-known international journals such as *Philosophy in Review, Deleuze Studies, Cultural Politics, Contemporary South Asia* and *Economic and Political Weekly*.

Tony See teaches in the National University of Singapore (NUS). His research interests include philosophy, critical theory and media studies. His current research interest is in exploring theories of subjectivity, with a focus on the intersections between Deleuze's idea of immanence and desire, and its resonances with the idea of Buddha-nature in Mahayana Buddhism. His previous publications include the book *Community Without Identity: The Ontology and Politics of Heidegger* (2009), and a number of articles such as 'Deleuze and Mahayana Buddhism' (2014), 'Deleuze and Ikeda' (2015) and 'Deleuze, Religion and Education' (2016).

Janae Sholtz is Associate Professor of Philosophy at Alvernia University. She has published articles in *PhiloSOPHIA: A Journal of Continental Feminism*. She has contributed chapters to *The Continuum Companion to Heidegger* edited by François Raffoul and Eric S. Nelson (2013) and *Between Deleuze and Foucault* edited by Daniel W. Smith, Thomas Nail and Nicolae Morar (forthcoming). She is the author of *The Invention of a People: Heidegger and Deleuze on Art and the Political* (2015) and co-editor of *Deleuze and the Schizoanalysis of Feminism* (2019). Sholtz has recently edited *French and Italian Stoicisms: From Sartre to Agamben* (2020).

Elizabeth Vasileva writes about ethics, radical politics and contemporary philosophy, being particularly inspired by Deleuze, Guattari, Braidotti and other new materialists. She is one of the organizers and lecturers at the Free University Brighton and Free University London, as well as a convenor of the Anarchist Studies Network.

Damian Ward Hey is a professor of literature and theory at Molloy College. He is the founder and EIC at *Stone Poetry Journal*.

Preface: Escaping Anthropocenity

Saswat Samay Das and Ananya Roy Pratihar

Pandemics breed *in-between* zones of natality while effecting gargantuan cycles of death and devastation. Yet the novelty of the current pandemic cannot be reduced to its paradoxical constituents. No doubt, in a nuanced manner every pandemic has signalled an ecological crisis. There is even a noteworthy range of interpretations holding out natural ecology as a palimpsest of anthropocentric exploitation. With the sheer encyclopaedic stockpile of such interpretations, in addition to those showing how Anthropocenity, instead of turning Spinozian ethics into praxis in light of the dense inter-relatedness between nature and earthlings, has manipulated and exploited the latter, throughout this volume the chapters ask where does the novelty of this outbreak lie in epistemic terms? And why is it necessary to link this outbreak and the whole history of the pandemic with Deleuze and Guattari's thinking?

While nature makes its grammatology perceptible to all its entities so they could live by nature by initiating a form of non-philosophical non-humanist engagement with it – the dynamics of *magic*, *occult* and *mysticism* have always shown a form of positive engagement with nature or the process of allying with or being escorted by nature – it is the natural yet double-pincered technicity of humans that expresses the problematics of their being. While technicity expresses human ability to treat nature as a therapeutic tool box, by putting it to repeated use the latter ends up engineering what Deleuze calls 'the semiotic regime', the plane of socio-symbolic displacement. To understand these workings of nature what is required is an intensive engagement with Deleuze and Guattari's thinking because this time the pandemic doesn't merely reflect its violent rejection of anthropocentric policies, rather the violence which nature has sparked off has a grammar similar to that of the violence that usually accompanies the capitalist exploitative reordering of ecology. The current pandemic only captures the viciousness of this repetition.

With current pandemics assailing the strata of our being, our private and public selves – sticking to our bodies, compelling us to master the methods of maintaining private hygiene, forcing us to embrace moral asceticism, keeping us confined to our domestic spaces, contaminating the palimpsestic body of the capital and even stultifying the public transportation, the very means of migration, movement and flow – our present volume mostly wields *eventuality* – one of Deleuze's several theoretical weapons in order to think through and register at the same time the multiple nuanced ways a (post)pandemic could be mapped out only to catch, albeit speculatively, the *new earth* and *new people* that Deleuze and Guattari so much hinted at.

Ironically, the 'normality' of this new normal lies in the nuanced violence it precipitates. This happens to be a violence that doesn't so much alter the organistic structuration of our bodies, but is directed at devastating the affectual smooth territoriality of our unconscious. As the biopolitical apparatuses of capture continue to implement their policies of lockdown to contain the pandemics, we are almost forced to become an organic bloc at odds with the de-conceptual reconstructing of our being. While contemporary philosophies restructure our beings, transforming us from instruments of mobilization to kinetic entities constituted by dynamics of *haecceities*, we are forced to revolve around our homes, slavishly sticking to the politically constructed and prescriptive understanding of the latter as a sacral territory where we experience real belongingness. Forcing a reinterpretation of ourselves in terms of the exclusive boundaries of our homes – given that the whole of the expanding middle class in urban locales stay in pigeon-holed quarters – the anthropocentric measures of implementing lockdowns lay the ground for the production of neurosis, paranoia and schizophrenia. However, the war on pandemics that our Institutions declare also gives them the liberty to keep our neuroses under expansive surveillance. This is a process that not only reduces our body to a networked play of divisional units, but ensures that we gradually start loving our state of neurosis rather than desiring to reclaim our originary schizoidical self. There is an uncanny parallel between the repressive measures our government undertakes to subdue pandemics and the ones it undertakes to quell other reactionary forces opposed to it. The violence which these events spark off goes on to reflect the strange intertwinement and interplay between the violence that the eco-sphere exercises through pandemics and that which anthropocentric governmental regimes exercise to contain it, reaffirming its hegemony over the rich vitalism of eco-systems and the public sphere. It may be argued that this restructuration of human society necessitates the emergence of new ways of existence by de-territorializing us from the capitalist networks and simultaneously re-territorializing us in the restrictive mobility of our domestic spheres. But is this what Deleuze and Guattari meant by de/re-territorialization? The chapters collected here attempt to address that.

The present global crisis requires our efforts for the creation of autonomous spaces empowered with a transformative potential. The unfolding catastrophe of geo-politics today requires fresh optics and new philosophical positioning, which we think Deleuzo-Guattarian thinking might offer. But focus should not be made on a structured sequential model of revolution, rather as revolutionaries we must try to exist in multiplicities and escape from such models because the aim is not to attain a goal. Rather the aim needs to be to find a new flow with spontaneous transformation. And it is this inscription of agency of transformation within events that makes the pandemical times stand pregnant with possibilities. And these are possibilities that could arrest the formation of post-pandemical capitalism and altogether wipe out the statist ideologies from triggering off a new world (dis)order.

Is Deleuze and Guattari's *becomings-multiple* the answer then? We argue that at this point we need to turn to Deleuze and Guattari's thinking that affords an exercise in creative violence, for it is only the creative violence of Deleuze and Guattari's thinking that could negate the *oedipality* of anthropocentric violence and build up an uncontrollable drive towards a rich 'non-human becoming' or what Guattari in *Chaosmosis* suggests to be 'new systems of valorization, a new taste for life, a new gentleness between the sexes, generations, ethnic groups, races'.

We suggest that violently opposing or revolting against the anthropocentrism may not be the best way to cancel or negate it as much as partaking of creative violence engendered by Deleuze and Guattari's thinking would be. And this collective partaking of creative violence tantamount to dwelling not merely in the non-spatial interstices or in-betweens of humanity but on the surfaces or limits of human experience will soon drive us into a state of unlearning all the anthropocentric codes, the mastery of which is required to be integral to socio-symbolic humanism in the first place. According to Andrew Culp, 'radical politics is all about attempting to identify those lines of flight which the state cannot prevent from escaping despite their potential to pose a threat to the existence of the former'. Culp puts forward this argument, for it is only these lines of flight that the state cannot figure out how to control that will eventually bring about the state's entropy or its re-territorialization around the natural kinship society in sync with the immanent patterns of nature. No doubt, it is necessary to identify lines of flight that the state cannot prevent from escaping not only because we could collectively embody them and become imperceptible to the state control mechanisms, but to give an effective shape to the micropolitical collectivistic desire for decisively de-territorializing from the current scenario. And this happens to be an act that demands exponentially generating such lines of flight. The only way one may do this is to exist in the socius one desires to de-territorialize from as a de-subjectivized, non-idententarian, non-facial and non-human becoming. And to exist in this state would mean ceaselessly and tirelessly finding out ways not to just creatively map the violent creativity of Deleuzo-Guattarian thinking, but to eternally trigger off processes of providing praxial turn to his thinking, which lays the ground for such existential becomings.

We argue that Deleuze's conceptualization of affective temporalities of life on earth that ranges from positioning onto-power as a pure potentia to disrupting the linearity of time and producing lines of flight is the only effective answer to anthropocentric agendas, which seems desirous in the current scenario to resuscitate itself by turning the new normal into mechanisms of generating profit. In fact, these potential lines of flight create cracks in the system of control; they reveal open spaces and experimental planes beyond the limits of what exists. The wide array of Deleuzo-Guattarian concepts may once again become the source for encountering the crisis caused by the pandemic. So, the collective desire at this moment ought to be to erect a platform to investigate in a variety of ways and perspectives the multiscalar eventuality of the pandemic, exposing a desire to explore new *unnatural alliances* that Deleuze and Guattari's philosophy offers to the post-pandemic new earth. Our book captures this collective desire to *become worthy of such events*.

SSD and ARP

Acknowledgements

We are immensely grateful to our contributors of this edited collection, many of whom struggled a lot in their personal spaces during the COVID-19 outbreak while giving the finest shape to the chapters. We are also indebted to Prof. Ian Buchanan, without whose support and guidance this book wouldn't have been possible. We also appreciate Jade Gordon at Bloomsbury who was always there with us from the very beginning of the publication process. We both would love to thank our young buddy and emerging scholar of Deleuze and Guattari Studies, Dipra Sarkhel, for helping us out through the editorial process.

The pain of the first and second waves of COVID-19 still hovers around us, and we are living with an incessant feeling of uncertainty even now. However, we are grateful to all those who have helped us endlessly in these trying times by giving us the space to work effortlessly on this edited volume.

Introduction

Paul Patton
Wuhan University

The pandemic

The year 2020 saw the emergence of the first truly global pandemic since the influenza outbreak in 1918–1919, in which the so-called Spanish flu infected roughly one third of the world's population and killed somewhere between 20 and 50 million people. The full cost of the COVID-19 pandemic is yet to be realized so it is unclear whether, purely in terms of the number of lives lost, it will be more or less severe than the flu pandemic in 1918–1919. As of the end of 2022 there were more than 659 million cases and over 6.6 million deaths worldwide.[1] The long-term consequences on the health of those infected continue to unfold and there is much still to be learned about the 'long Covid' suffered by some. The broader ramifications of the pandemic continue to affect the lives of individuals, the health of economies, the standing of governments and the global political order in ways that are only beginning to become apparent. All indications are that this will be an event that marks a significant break with the past on a number of levels: epidemiological, economic, social, political and geopolitical.

At its most basic level, the COVID-19 pandemic involved the transmission of a new coronavirus, SARS-CoV-2, in human populations that had no prior experience of this particular pathogen and hence no bodily immunity to its effects. Importantly, the SARS-CoV-2 genome was mapped and published within weeks of its appearance. Genomic sequencing allows the identification of variations in the genetic code of the virus and, since these occur with considerable regularity, scientists can use them to track the movements of the virus around the world. The precise origins of this virus and the pathway that led it to infect people in the Chinese city of Wuhan have not been established and may never be known with any certainty. In part, this is because argument over the source or sources of the virus has become politicized to the extent that research into its origins has become a significant element of the pandemic as a geopolitical event. The current consensus is that it is a virus that existed in bats and that migrated to human beings, possibly by way of an intermediate animal species. Because markets where such animals are sold involved close proximity with many people, it was initially thought that SARS-CoV-2 may have first infected human beings at the Huanan Seafood Wholesale Market in Wuhan. However, while the majority of the first cases of infection that appeared in December 2019 had some connection to the Huanan market, others did not. So the market may not have been the source of the virus in human populations but rather the environment that first enabled it to be transmitted widely among human hosts. Once established in Wuhan in January 2020, the virus quickly spread throughout China, parts of Southeast Asia, Iran and Western Europe before it began to spread in the United States in March. On 11 March 2020, the World Health Organization declared the spread of SARS-CoV-2 to be a pandemic.

This is not the first time that a virus has migrated from an animal species to humans, nor will it be the last. Recent outbreaks as a result of inter-species transmission include varieties of Swine fever, Ebola virus, Bird flu and Hendra virus, to name but a few. However, none of these had the same combination of virulence and transmissibility as SARS-CoV-2. This would have enabled them to spread as far and as quickly throughout the human population as SARS-CoV-2 has been able to do. This virus belongs to a family of coronaviruses, so-called because of the spike proteins on the exterior of the virus that present a crown-like visual appearance. Other members of this family cause mild symptoms associated with the common cold. However some, such as SARS-1, also thought to have come from bats, produce more serious symptoms of the kind associated with COVID-19, including fever, dry cough, shortness of breath and sometimes fatal pneumonia. The SARS-1 epidemic in 2003 lasted about eight months and spread to around thirty countries, infecting around eight and half thousand people of whom 916 died.[2] The case fatality rate of SARS-1 was around 10.9 per cent, which is far less deadly than viruses such as Ebola that can reach a case fatality rate around 80 to 90 per cent, but deadly enough to make it difficult for the virus to spread widely: those affected die too quickly. SARS-CoV-2 does not have this problem. Estimates of its case fatality rate are around 0.5 to 1.2 per cent, which is ten times that of ordinary influenza but still ten times less than SARS-1.[3] For this reason, along with other features of the virus that affect its transmissibility, SARS-CoV-2 is a greater threat to human populations than SARS-1. A further distinguishing feature of COVID-19 is the fact that patients are infectious before they become symptomatic, which makes it much more difficult to control the spread of the disease. The proliferation of variants of SARS-CoV-2 also makes it difficult to stabilize by means of vaccines.

Thinking through the pandemic event

The chapters collected in this volume draw on aspects of Deleuze's philosophy, for the most part but not exclusively his work with Guattari. They also draw on the extensive secondary literature on Deleuze and the work of a range of contemporary thinkers, including New Materialist and feminist authors such as Barad, Bennett and Braidotti, theorists of biopolitics such as Agamben, Esposito, along with a number of other French philosophers such as Badiou, Derrida, Foucault, Nancy and Latour. For example, Janae Sholtz (Chapter 5) suggests that, in contrast to the philosophical tradition that opposes an active, free and independent subject to an inert or mechanical realm of nature, the New Materialist understanding of matter as dynamic provides a more helpful perspective in which to think through the entanglements of viral and human bodies. Several contributors take up the concept of biopolitics as introduced by Foucault and developed by others including Esposito and Agamben. More than one of the contributors makes use of Derrida's concept of 'autoimmunity', which has immediate application to the COVID-19 pandemic: a major cause of death during the first wave of infection was the 'cytokine storm' produced by the immune system's own response to infection. Clayton Crockett (Chapter 1) makes the point that it is the human body's own 'autoimmunity' that kills it in the case of viral infection: 'There is no community without auto-immunity, just as there is no organism that is not exposed to death precisely by virtue of its ability to be alive' (Crockett p. 13). Taken together, these chapters address a range of issues surrounding the nature of the pandemic, along with its direct as well as indirect social, cultural, economic and political effects. A recurrent theme is the manner in which the spread of the SARS-CoV-2 virus disrupted habitual patterns and allowed for the emergence of new ways of thinking, acting and being. A key focus for several chapters is Deleuze's concept of the event and its relevance for understanding the pandemic.

The nature of events was a recurrent concern in Deleuze's work, as it was for many of the cohort of French philosophers to which he belonged. Deleuze described this concern with the nature of events as a focus on the question of 'the emergence of the new'.[4] What he meant by this was that the philosophers of his generation with whom he identified such as Châtelet, Lyotard and Foucault among others were all profoundly historical thinkers, less concerned with timeless or universal conditions of possibility than with the historically specific conditions of what actually happens. In the homage that he wrote after Deleuze's death in 1995, Derrida described him as more than anything else 'the thinker of the event'.[5] Derrida also aligned himself with the focus on the nature of events and the emergence of the new shared by the cohort that became known as 'poststructuralist' philosophers.

The COVID-19 pandemic is an extremely complex event, at once virological, epidemiological and medical, but also economic and geopolitical. The pandemic event unfolds in all of these dimensions, evolving and mutating as a consequence of interactions between the different dimensions or layers of the event. At every level, the pandemic is entangled in power relations between individuals, institutions, states and species that make it a profoundly political event.[6] While the virological and epidemiological dimensions of the event are not new, the consequences of a global pandemic under the prevailing economic and geopolitical conditions are entirely novel. Following Deleuze's remarks about the ethics of events, the COVID-19 pandemic poses a problem for philosophical and ethical reflection, namely how to counteractualize or to become worthy of this event.

Francisco J. Alcalá's 'Thinking the COVID-19 as an Event' (Chapter 12) directly confronts the pandemic with what he notes is regarded by Deleuze as a 'core notion of his thought' (Alcalá p. 172). He retraces the outlines in *Difference and Repetition* of Deleuze's concept of the event as a 'redistribution of the constitutive powers of reality at the transcendental level' before outlining a conception of the pandemic in Deleuzian terms. Among the many features of the pandemic that make it susceptible to analysis in Deleuzian terms, he singles out the manner in which the novelty of the virus establishes a new form of equality in which everyone is potentially a subject of contagion. This is the new 'milieu of immanence' on which the pandemic erupts. In keeping with the 'horizontality' of contagion as a relation that cuts across the hierarchies of the natural world, the pandemic exposes the contingency and mutability of the hierarchies that define our social world. As such, for Alcalá, as for several other contributors, the pandemic is not entirely a negative phenomenon but one that 'makes us experience the nonsense of a large part of the hierarchies on which our routines, movements, relationships, expectations and, in the end, our lives are based' (Alcalá p. 177). In these terms, becoming equal to the pandemic event is a matter of drawing the lesson of universal susceptibility to contagion 'by establishing international solidarity agreements, effective public policies and interpersonal care networks' (Alcalá p. 180). If there are lessons of resistance to be drawn, these should not be directed at state efforts to contain the pandemic and to protect the vulnerable but rather at the reluctance to do so in the name of protecting an impersonal and inhumane economy, and at the purveyors of 'post-truth' and conspiracy theories seeking to profit from the proliferation of information about the pandemic and its causes. For Alcalá, counter-effectuation of the pandemic event should involve the promotion of a non-dogmatic 'scientific and humanist culture focused on the formation of problems' (Alcalá p. 181).

Kyle Novak's 'On the Difference Between Morality and Ethics in the New Normal: Gilles Deleuze's Spinozist Ethics in the Context of COVID-19' (Chapter 10) provides a quite different ethical response to the pandemic. He draws on the contrast that Deleuze develops in his work on Spinoza between morality and ethics in order to argue that an 'ethical response to the COVID-19 pandemic should resist the moralizing of the New Normal and instead have an immanent focus on what is happening to us' (Novak p. 139). Novak explains the difference between these two approaches in terms of the distinction between the moral aspiration to pass judgement and the ethical aspiration to understand what is happening. He points out that this distinction also aligns with Spinoza's contrast between the sad passions that accompany our transition to lesser states of power and the joyful passions that accompany our transition to higher states of power. In these terms, Novak proposes a response not so much to the pandemic as to the measures instigated in response, the so-called 'New Normal', asking to what extent these serve to increase or to decrease our power of acting. His response is unambiguously critical. For many, especially the most vulnerable members of society, these measures have led to little more than 'a semblance of life' (Novak p. 150). Novak draws on Bartleby's noncommittal act of refusal in suggesting that the appropriate response to moralizing injunctions to wear a mask, stay home or get vaccinated should be simply 'I would prefer not to' (Novak p. 150).

Yet another response is outlined in Jernej Markelj's 'The Ethics of Paranoia: How to Become Worthy of COVID-19' (Chapter 11), which draws on Deleuze's earlier work including his analysis of ressentiment in *Nietzsche and Philosophy*, the stoic ethics of the event in *Logic of Sense* and the theory of social and individual desire developed with Guattari in *Anti-Oedipus*. The result is a cogent analysis of the effect of the SARS-CoV-2 pandemic within the context of the libidinal dynamic of late capitalism. Markelj argues that by interrupting the availability of labour along with the flows of goods and services, COVID-19 and the measures imposed to slow its inexorable spread further encourage the tendency towards paranoia that is endemic to capitalist society. Given the fragmentation of social orders of belief and behaviour that is both a product of the decoding and deterritorializing tendency of capitalism and reinforced by digital technology that divides populations into increasingly isolated echo chambers of opinion, paranoia becomes a feature of ever smaller and more culturally diverse segments. However, rather than condemning this state of affairs, Markelj uses Deleuze's analysis in *Nietzsche and Philosophy* of the positive effect of *ressentiment* on the development of human thought and sentiment to take the counter-intuitive position of asking what we might gain from the varieties of Covid-induced paranoia. He suggests that another way to respond to Deleuze's injunction in *Logic of Sense* to become worthy of the events that befall us might be 'to push beyond our *ressentiment*, acquiescence and all the "*if only*'s" that this pandemic has inspired, and invent ways of living that will allow us to face its consequences with lightness or even laughter' (Markelj p. 167).

The 'evental' nature of the virus and the viral nature of events

Many of the chapters collected here draw on the rich array of novel philosophical concepts developed in Deleuze and Guattari's *A Thousand Plateaus*, to elucidate particular aspects of the COVID-19 pandemic. One reason why these concepts are especially useful in relation to this viral pandemic lies in the fundamentally viral character of Nature as described by Deleuze and Guattari. As Brent Adkins (Chapter 3) notes, 'Viruses form an important touchstone throughout *A Thousand Plateaus*' (Adkins p. 46). He points to the manner in which Deleuze and Guattari's concepts of Nature and micropolitics are viral through and through. In *Dialogues*, Deleuze and Parnet comment on the tendency in contemporary science to be less concerned with discovering invariant structures than with retracing the course of singular, incorporeal events that are effected in bodies and states of affairs. They give the example of the event of reproduction or replication 'which happens in a gel, but also in an epidemic or in a news item'.[7] Their point is that viral reproduction is a complex, ongoing event that includes variation as well as repetition in the structure of the genome. This is true of literal as well as informational viruses. These are not objects with stable essential properties so much as events that unfold in particular ways as a consequence of the nature of the host as much as that of the viral material introduced. As John Dupré and Stephan Guttinger point out, the life-cycle of a given virus

> should not be understood as some sort of material thing or as a mere succession of different states of one material thing that gives the cycle its unity. Rather, the process of the cycle as a whole is the virus. And the viral life-cycle is one of the many processes that may come together to form yet another stable pattern to which we usually refer as 'organism'.[8]

There are therefore profound resonances between the 'evental' nature of the virus and the viral nature of events as Deleuze and Guattari describe them. On their account, Nature is fundamentally viral. It proceeds through becomings and across rhizomatic connections between heterogenous elements that initiate new forms of deterritorialization and reterritorialization.

Damian Ward Hey's schizo-essay 'Deleuze and Guattari, The Pandemic, the Trump Presidency and the Schizo-Analytic Essay Machine' (Chapter 7) points out that the structure of academic commentary is also viral in the manner in which it uses material from the object of commentary, the host, along with material gleaned from other commentary and information about the object in order to 'form its own body which then spreads through language to the brain which replicates it either in speaking or in writing perhaps producing mutations, new viral forms' (Hey p. 101). For Hey, the viral dimension of Nature is also manifest in the political field. He suggests that the Trump presidency, which overlapped with the COVID-19 pandemic and contributed through inaction to the severity of its effects in the United States, was itself a kind of virus that infected the body politic. Trumpism was at once parasitic on the organs of government and disruptive of the body politic by virtue of the manner in which it refused to follow many of the unwritten conventions that allow the system to work. The rhizomatic character of Trumpism and its roots in disaffection among those whose world had been deterritorialized by the effects of the same global capitalism on which Trump depended are no doubt among the reasons why many commentators compared it to fascism.

Clayton Crockett's 'Toward an Epidemiology of Morals' (Chapter 1) mobilizes a number of viral concepts from *A Thousand Plateaus* in discussing the implications of the current pandemic, including the rhizomatic relationships that human beings form with other animals by virtue of cross-species viral transmission, the deterritorialization of human bodies and human societies effected by viral pandemics, and the ways in which viruses function as a war-machine that deterritorializes existing social and political assemblages: 'We need to think and comprehend the pandemic more rhizomatically, to see how the spread of the virus consists in not only a devastating illness but also a nomadic war machine that is deterritorializing the globe, creating new assemblages, alliances, and pandemic solidarities' (Crockett p. 20)

The virus as war machine is also central to Brent Adkins' argument in '*Obscura Sacrificia*: Covid and Neoliberalism' (Chapter 3) that the COVID-19 pandemic involves a conflict between the viral war machine and that of neoliberal capitalism. He develops an elegant analogy between this conflict and the ancient Greek story of the conflict between Agamemnon's fleet and the offended goddess Artemis, which also involved a collision between two war machines. Just as the conflict between the Greeks and the goddess was only resolved through the sacrifice of Agamemnon's daughter Iphigenia, so the conflict between the pandemic and the economic needs of neoliberal capitalism demanded sacrifice, whether of the aged or otherwise vulnerable segments of the population most at risk in the campaign to achieve herd immunity, or of those lower paid workers employed in so-called essential work who were unable to work from home or not work at all during the pandemic: 'Neoliberal capitalism is a war machine that exposes its suicidal tendencies when confronted by the war machine of a global pandemic as each tries to envelop the other' (Adkins p. 51).

Emine Görgül's 'Regimes of Exclusion and Control: Politics of Modern Space and Its Role in the Immunization and Pandemics' (Chapter 8) points to the long history of interaction between architecture and medicine in support of its central claim that architecture has long been 'a crucial component and a critical player in immunization and biopolitics' (Görgül p. 106). By pointing to elements of this history such as the ancient Roman *Asklepios* that served as a precursor of modern hospital architecture, she indirectly challenges the focus on European modernity as the beginnings of biopolitics. She also notes Deleuze and Guattari's reliance on viral processes of contagion in their accounts of the constitution and transformation of assemblages and draws a connection between the different ways in which deterritorialization and reterritorialization can impact on a body and the forms of autoimmunity that can become fatal for the host body. In recent architectural history, she refers to the example of the *Märkisches Viertel* in Berlin that was designed and built in the 1960s as a showpiece of public housing before becoming a site of radical activism and opposition to the state.

Societies of control and beyond

Several of the chapters in this volume take their point of departure from Deleuze's 'Postscript on Societies of Control'. Francisco J. Alcalá (Chapter 12) suggests that state responses to the pandemic confirm at every point Deleuze's description of societies of control: 'the empire of digital numbers [*chiffre*] that determine access to information, the control mechanisms that determine at every moment the position of an individual in an open environment, or Félix Guattari's fantasy of an electronic card that would allow us to move freely by opening a series of barriers ... until it was subject to temporary or permanent restrictions' (Alcalá p. 178). Other contributors such as Brad Evans and Chantal Meza seek to update the diagnosis of Deleuze's essay by drawing attention to ways in which twenty-first century bio-power takes the form of an accelerated 'technologization of life':

> We are, in short, in a condition today that is truly *Beyond Control* as the triumph of the technical imagination is writ large as it seeks to colonize every creative expression, every thought, every projection, every concern; making a nomadism of technological abstraction fully possibly, while denying the human any autonomy to freely roam or to even imagine some viable escape (especially intellectual) (Evans and Meza pp. 25–26).

In 'Beyond Control: Technology, Post-Faciality and the Dance of the Abstract' (Chapter 2), Evans and Meza point to the possibilities of an artistic and poetic imagination as a source of resistance to the contemporary 'global techno-theodicy' (Evans and Meza p. 24). They also suggest that the widespread rapid acceptance of masking in societies that had recently been stridently opposed to the veil shows the obsolescence of the Abstract Machine of Faciality – discussed in Plateau 5, '587 B.C.–A.D. 70: On Several Regimes of Signs' in *A Thousand Plateaus* – in favour of a new form of power whose target is the mind rather than the body.

Virgilio A. Rivas (Chapter 9) notes the ways in which facial recognition technology contributes to a new form of 'faciality' that operates in tandem with the ubiquitous masking of the population and reduces the human face to the eyes visible above the mask. He takes Deleuze's 'Societies of Control' essay as the point of departure for reflections on the social, technological and political changes that were already underway before being exacerbated by the pandemic. Invoking the failed becoming-animal of Kafka's Gregor Samsa, Rivas points to the emergence of a new kind of techno-human assemblage that is the effect not only of the becoming-animal in relation to the virus, if indeed it is an animal, but also of the incorporation of AI-driven technology along with the range of social measures intended to curb the spread of the virus. Together these define 'the new normal' and the emergence of what might be called a contaminated people. The fate of such a people in a world increasingly threatened with ecological as well as virological and algorithmic catastrophe remains to be determined.

The connection between technologies of communication and surveillance and the further development of societies of control also provides the point of departure for Tony See Sin Heng's exploration in 'The Task of Thinking in The Age of Biopolitics: Between Heidegger and Deleuze' (Chapter 4) of the biopolitical dimension of the pandemic. See Sin Heng draws on Giorgio Agamben's much discussed argument that State responses to the pandemic are as much about establishing a permanent state of exception as they are about public health, as well as Heidegger's delineation of the technological frame of modern thought, in order to pursue Deleuze's question of the possibility of thinking outside or beyond the form of State-thought. How is such thinking possible, See Sin Heng asks: 'The task of thinking is yet to be complete and maybe, just maybe, the rise of biopolitics in the midst of this COVID-19 global pandemic is "the outside" that will force us to take up the task of thinking.' (See Sin Heng p. 63).

Covid, culture and community

A final cluster of chapters in this volume relate to what we might call cultural dimensions of the pandemic, its impact on people's understanding of the world and the communities in which they live. Janae Sholtz's 'Post-Covid Communities: Immanent Engagements and Intersectional Transversality' (Chapter 5) argues that the lessons to be drawn from the COVID-19 pandemic include the need to rethink 'the parameters of community and individuality' in order to foster 'a deeper awareness of our immanent immersive engagements' (Sholtz p. 65). Sholtz argues that political analysis of the pandemic and its effects can benefit from Deleuze and Guattari's approach to transversality and their appreciation of the ways in which molecular becomings both feed into and are conditioned by molar social and political identities: 'We need a way of thinking transversal relations, which attune us to how our "selves" are formed and generated through immersive intra-actions, *along with* intersectional approaches that directly confront systems of oppression' (Sholtz p. 72). Writing from the perspective of an American experience of the pandemic and its effects on communities, she suggests that this new way of thinking implies an affective transformation in the ways that 'we' relate to others. This implies nothing less than a new form of love that Sholtz proposes to understand in the light of Guattari's call in *Chaosmosis* to create 'new systems of valorization, a new taste for life, a new gentleness between the sexes, generations, ethnic groups, races' (cited Sholtz p. 74).

Elizabeth Vasileva's 'A Cartography of Mutual Aid Groups in Brighton' (Chapter 13) also discusses the reconfiguration of community under the conditions imposed by Covid. Hers is the only chapter that takes up these issues from a social science perspective, outlining a Deleuze and Guattari inspired cartography of the mutual aid groups that sprang up in the English seaside town of Brighton during lockdown. At its peak, Brighton had more than eighty mutual aid groups entirely staffed and run by volunteers, including retirees and others involuntarily furloughed from their employment. These groups formed a rhizomatic network with online presence and applications developed for specific purposes such as ordering food or furniture. Vasileva maps key elements of the environmental, social and mental ecology of Brighton that help to explain this phenomenon. These groups provided a powerful demonstration of the capacity for self-organization and the possibility of large-scale reterritorialization of desire. Their lateral rather than hierarchical relationship to the recipients of aid pointed to the possibility of different kinds of social relationship and a different kind of community emerging from the socially and economically diverse population of Brighton and surrounding regions. Vasileva shows how the social history and predisposition to forms of community action, the space opened by the removal of the usual constraints on social life, and the relative lack of institutional actors able to respond to social needs allowed ordinary people to discover or rediscover the 'efficiency and joyfulness of self-organization' (Vasileva p. 191).

Patricia Pisters' 'The Limits of Perception: Knights of Narcotics, Nonhuman Aesthetics and the Psychedelic Revival' (Chapter 6) explores the lessons of Deleuze and Guattari's experimental philosophy and Deleuze's philosophy of cinema for making sense of the contemporary revival of interest in psychedelic substances. While this does not involve the kind of counter-cultural movement that accompanied the psychedelic phenomena of the 1960s, it shares with that counter-culture, and with earlier forms of experimentation, an interest in the aesthetic consequences of using psychedelic substances. When Deleuze and Guattari suggest that drugs change perceptions of the world, even on the part of non-users,[9] they draw attention to the relationship between experimental art and experimentation with psychedelics: both are ways in which human sensibility and its aesthetic relation to the world can be transformed. Pisters suggests that Deleuze finds a parallel concern on the part of some experimental filmmakers, for whom the camera and editing techniques offer a means to produce a 'nonhuman perception that at its limits of intensity becomes a means to create a psychedelic aesthetic experience with different, artistic and technological means' (Pisters p. 84). The pandemic too disrupts our habituated ways of acting in ways that may lead to a reconfiguration of our aesthetic relation to the world. The experience of life less dominated by work and the imperative to produce may in turn encourage new ethical relations and new forms of belief in the world.

These brief snapshots of the chapters hardly do justice to the richness of this book. So too is the thematic grouping above no more than one way of relating the diverse contents of these extraordinary chapters. It contains no instruction regarding the order in which they should be read, which should rather be understood on the model of an album that one samples in pursuit of a particular interest or desire. However you read it, this book will enrich your understanding of the pandemic and open up new perspectives on the philosophy of Deleuze and Guattari.

Notes

1 Data from the Johns Hopkins University Coronavirus Resource Center at https://coronavirus.jhu.edu/map.html (last accessed 22 July 2022).
2 Nicholas A. Christakis, *Apollo's Arrow: The profound effect and enduring impact of coronavirus on the way we live*, New York: Little, Brown and Spark, 2020, 92.
3 Christakis, *Apollo's Arrow*, 96.
4 Gilles Deleuze, *Negotiations 1972–1990*, trans. Martin Joughin, New York: Columbia University Press, 1995, 86.
5 Jacques Derrida, 'I'm Going to Have to Wander All Alone', in Pascale-Ann Brault and Michael Naas, trans. and eds., *The Work of Mourning*, Chicago: University of Chicago Press, 2001, 189–196.
6 Paul Patton, 'In what sense is the Corona phenomenon *political*?' in Pegah Mossleh ed. *Corona Phenomenon. Philosophical and Political Questions*, Leiden and Boston: Brill, 2022, 125–132.
7 Gilles Deleuze and Claire Parnet, *Dialogues II*, trans. Hugh Tomlinson and Barbara Habberjam, London: Athlone Press 2002, 67.
8 John Dupré and Stephan Guttinger, 'Viruses as living processes', *Studies in History and Philosophy of Biological and Biomedical Sciences*, 59, 2016, 109–116.
9 Gilles Deleuze and Félix Guattari, *A Thousand Plateaus: Capitalism and Schizophrenia*, trans. Brian Massumi, Minneapolis: University of Minnesota Press, 1987, 248.

1

Toward an Epidemiology of Morals

Clayton Crockett

This chapter develops an 'epidemiology of morals' based on *A Thousand Plateaus*, where the *virus* is an indication of the absolute deterritorialization of Earth, giving us a glimpse of a new Nomos of the Earth beyond neoliberal global capitalism. A virus is a quasi-living parasite upon life, but we cannot properly assign what is life and what is not from the perspective of the virus. It is a quasi-organic and quasi-inorganic form of life that consists of an abstract replication machine. This machine self-replicates within its host and creates destructive assemblages with and against the immune system of its bearer. Although vaccines are a key component in human resistance against viruses, we also need means of comprehending how they enable new forms of solidarity, and potentially reshape our earth.

What can a virus do?

Virus is derived from the Latin word for poison due to its effect on humans and other animals. Virology emerged at the end of the nineteenth century as a Russian (Dmitri Ivanovsky) and a Dutch (Martinus Beijerinck) scientist searched for an agent that causes the tobacco mosaic disease. It was Beijerinck who realized that the disease agent was not a bacterium, but a new kind of existent. A virus exists at the edge of the living and the nonliving. It is a form of quasi-organic life because it contains genetic material (DNA or RNA) but it does not have a metabolism or a cell structure. Viruses appear to have evolved from bacteria and they are extremely small in relation to bacteria, not to mention multicellular organisms. They could not be 'seen' until the development of electron microscopes in the twentieth century.

A virus is a membrane that contains genetic material within it. It is a parasite that can only truly exist within a host cell and its function is replication. It possesses protuberances or spikes to fit into receptor cells of the host organism. Once the virus enters the cell it folds and refolds upon itself and eventually fuses with the cell. The genes of the virus penetrate the nucleus of the cell and displace the cell's genes and instruct the cells to produce viral proteins. The virus thus self-replicates, producing millions of copies of itself inside a cell that then explodes, transmitting them to other cells in a swarm.

Once a virus successfully self-replicates and invades surrounding cells, the body's immune system gears up to fight it. Sometimes the body is rendered susceptible to serious or even fatal infections, and other times the intensity of the body's own immune system causes the illness to become more destructive. Often the respiratory tract is stripped of vital epithelial cells by the infection, which leaves it and the lungs more vulnerable to attack by viral pneumonia.

When the virus infection spreads, the immune system responds with inflammation that creates redness, heat and swelling at the site of the infection, in an attempt to contain it. Alternatively, the immune system may inflame the entire body with a fever in an attempt to kill off the invading cells. As one book explains, 'the actual process of inflammation involves the release of certain white blood cells of proteins called "cytokines"'.[1] These cytokines are what generally cause the toxic effects of pain and suffering we associate with an illness that makes us sick.

In cases of acute viral infection the ultimate struggle occurs in the lungs, where the virus, the cytokines and pneumonia meet in the form of Acute Respiratory Distress Syndrome (ARDS). Here the immune systems follows the virus into the lungs and unleashes its 'killer T cells', which targets the body's own infected cells. The all-out war that results kills the virus and sometimes the patient in a 'cytokine storm', 'a desperate attack using every lethal weapon the body possesses'. Although the infection is caused by the virus, the ARDS results from the immune system's own toxins that create 'a burn inside the lungs . . . scorching the tissue'.[2] This autoimmune response recalls the famous line uttered by an American Major during the Vietnam War, as reported by Peter Arnett: 'It became necessary to destroy the town to save it.'

Both influenza and SARS-CoV-2 are RNA viruses, which replicate and spread much more rapidly than DNA viruses. Both influenza and SARS-CoV-2, or the COVID-19 coronavirus, usually kill people as a result of ARDS. The coronavirus mutates much more slowly compared with the influenza virus, but it is so communicable due to its infectious nature that these mutations have made it capable of avoiding the vaccines that have already been deployed against it.[3] This word coronavirus refers to its morphology, which appears like a crown, and its shape and behaviour suggest what Deleuze calls a 'crowned anarchy' in *Difference and Repetition*. Here is an intensity 'that is suspect only because it seems to rush headlong into suicide'. In fact, this suicide rush is a form of madness: 'it proposes mad distribution – instantaneous, nomadic distribution, crowned anarchy or difference'.[4] The anarchic difference that is generated by COVID-19's mad distribution is destructive to human life and social order; however, in a strange way its behaviour opens up the possibility to glimpse new kinds of intensities, new forms of deterritorialization, new solidarities and even new kinds of kin.

Auto-immunity

About a century ago, another pandemic struck the world that was much more devastating and deadly than our current one. In some ways, the COVID-19 virus is a strange repetition of the so-called Spanish influenza pandemic of 1918. Of course, its death count is far lower, at least so far, but it has spread as far and as fast as that global pandemic. We do not know for certain where the influenza virus began, although it has been speculated that it originated in the United States in a milder form, then spread across the world. It became much more deadly as a result of a mutation and spread among troops who were being demobilized from the Great War. The total number of deaths was more than 50 million people, and this is a somewhat low estimate. The influenza virus itself was not identified until long after the pandemic, but it was a strain of H1N1 that crossed the boundary from birds to humans.[5]

Due to the close proximity of humans and other domesticated animals to each other as a result of the development of agriculture, many new diseases have spread, often as a result of a lack of fresh water. These diseases include bacterial and viral killing assemblages, and they are met by the body's incredibly powerful immune system. In fact, it is the immune system that often causes death, rather than the disease itself.

According to Jacques Derrida, this physiological auto-immunity also applies to human society. As he analyses religion in his essay 'Faith and Knowledge', Derrida posits an 'excess above and beyond the living, whose life only has absolute value by being worth more than life, more than itself'. This excessive status of life paradoxically threatens the living organism, because it 'opens the space of death that is linked to the automaton ... in other words, to the dimensions of auto-immune and self-sacrificial supplementarity'.[6] There is no community without auto-immunity, just as there is no organism that is not exposed to death precisely by virtue of its ability to be alive.

In terms of a viral infection, the auto-immunity is deadly due to its going into overdrive, a desperate death drive that destroys the organism in its attempt to annihilate the attacker. This is also the political logic of the war against terrorism that broke out in the wake of the terrorist attacks of September 11, 2001. The Bush administration was going to destroy the American way of life in order to save it, to give up civil liberties in order to preserve them, to defeat the enemy by going to such extremes that it would sacrifice American democracy.

Every state takes steps to protect itself, and it appeals to law or right to justify these protections, while enforcing them with violence. Every society was forced to shut down at least partially as the COVID-19 virus spread around the world in early 2020. Some of these measures were rational and many were not. The most schizophrenic response was that of the United States, which politicized the response to the virus to such an extent it created a society almost at war with itself: wearing masks or getting vaccinated was a deprivation of liberty rather than a medically responsible action for many people. The president, Donald Trump, encouraged and inflamed these responses in a desperate and failed attempt to gain re-election. These microscopic viruses acted as 'terror agents' upon the American people beyond their deadly bio-medical effects.

As Derrida states in an interview after 9/11, the 'relationship between earth, *terra*, territory, and terror has changed, and it is necessary to know that this is because of knowledge, that is, because of technoscience'.[7] In many ways, the American and to some extent the European response was to want to assimilate these attacks and this 'war on terror' to an older and more heroic understanding of war; but that is impossible. Why? Because of the question of scale, which has become much smaller, much more minor: 'nanotechnologies of all sorts are so much more powerful and invisible, uncontrollable, capable of creeping in everywhere. They are the micrological rivals of microbes and bacteria', even as we face real microbes in our struggle to survive in a twenty-first century postmodern landscape.[8]

In some ways, it's as though Derrida were citing Deleuze's 1992 'Postscript on the Societies of Control' in this interview from 2003. These new micro-technologies of control are both maintained and threatened by these multitudes of nanotechnologies, computer viruses and real viruses. The 'coils of the serpent' bind us ever more tightly to the capitalist machine, which has used the enormous drop in production caused by the pandemic to accelerate the transfer of wealth from poor to rich that has been underway since at least the 1970s.[9]

At the same time, the existence of the virus attests to a new model of evolution, one that is inherently rhizomatic. In the Introduction to *A Thousand Plateaus*, Deleuze and Guattari cite Rémy Chauvin, who suggests that we consider an '*apparallel evolution* of two beings that have absolutely nothing to do with each other'.[10] Our typical model of evolution follows a line of descent that constitutes a tree. However, under certain conditions, a virus can connect to germ cells and transmit itself as the cellular gene of a complex species. Here evolution occurs as a result of the heterogeneous or horizontal genetic transfer of already differentiated lines that leap across species in a rhizomatic fashion. The rhizome is the newer model of evolution, and the virus is a crucial component of this new image of thought. According to Deleuze and Guattari, 'we form a rhizome with our viruses, or rather our viruses cause us to form a rhizome with other animals'.[11]

Rather than adopting the perspective of our bodily immune system in its war against viruses, we need to appreciate how viruses themselves make us who we are. Genuine becomings are not merely genealogical descendences that are inherited characteristics. Rather, we must 'always look for the molecular, or even submolecular, particle with which we are allied. We evolve and die more from our polymorphous and rhizomatic flus than from hereditary diseases'.[12] What would it mean to ally ourselves with our viruses as opposed to our immune systems? What strange assemblages and new solidarities might result?

What is a body without organs?

The organs are the ultimate target of the virus: the lungs, the brain, the heart. These organs work organizationally and teleologically, protecting and preserving the body from harm; which, at the same time, by taking such extreme steps to save it, often destroys the patient. The organs work inside a person and keep them alive by keeping invaders out, despite the impossibility of establishing a boundary that would be impermeable and impenetrable to the outside.

In *A Thousand Plateaus*, specifically their chapter on 'The Geology of Morals', Deleuze and Guattari ground this body without organs in the earth. They cite Arthur Conan Doyle in explaining that the earth 'is a body without organs' that is 'permeated by unformed, unstable matters, by flows in all directions, by free intensities or nomadic singularities, by mad or transitory particles'.[13] They want to celebrate these aspects of the earth, while at the same time attending to the complex process of stratification that occurs along with it. Even as the body gets organized into strata, the virus appears as a 'free intensity' or 'mad particle' that threatens and exceeds it.

We stratify our bodies and our ideas according to what gets legislated as healthy in contemporary neoliberal terms. Our body becomes a state that must be maintained and defended against all invaders at any cost. This good sense of the healthy body is accomplished by means of what Deleuze and Guattari call a 'double articulation. Articulate twice, B-A, BA'. The first articulation, B-A, creates 'metastable molecular or quasi-molecular units' and establishes a connection by associating one term or phenomena with another.[14] The second articulation, BA, conjoins the two together to form a functional stable order that appears natural and given. We approach the body from the standpoint of the second articulation, already persuaded of the primacy of the stratified, segmented body that functions with its organs according to the telos of an organization.

The forms and substances of the body generate a code and a territory. The territory is the area that is occupied by this or that body, while the code represents the genetic program that makes it work. Here Deleuze and Guattari are ostensibly talking about geological strata, but they are also employing biological terms in their incredibly abstract analysis. I am appropriating their discussion of geology for the more specific purposes of biology and virology, because what they identify as the processes of free intensities and nomadic singularities applies very aptly to a virus. The virus lacks the metabolism and therefore the organization of bodies. It is a machinic assemblage that self-replicates at the edge of life, inserting itself within the gap between the living and the nonliving.

There is no coding without decoding, in genetic and epigenetic terms. In their discussion of codes and coding, Deleuze and Guattari note that 'as soon as it is recognized that a code is inseparable from a process of decoding that is inherent in it, the problem receives a new formulation. There is no genetics without "genetic drift"'.[15] Every code possesses a supplement that is available for free variation, which is a different kind of double articulation because here the second articulation is left open for transfer and variation. This is how evolution works, by means of surplus or excess.

In addition to genetic mutation, that according to sexual reproduction of multicellular organisms, bacteria reproduce by asexual division or mitosis. In many ways, this process is more simple than the complex meiosis of eukaryotic organisms, but it allows bacteria to reproduce much more quickly, and to accomplish what is called horizontal gene transfers. Horizontal gene transfers work by altering a cell with the introduction of new genetic material to create new forms of a species. These transfers also occur in eurkaryotes, which are nucleated cells, along with the multicellular organisms that they compose, but it is less well known or studied compared with sexual reproduction via gametes.

The virus, however, reproduces by introducing its own genetic material (RNA or DNA) and hijacking a cell's metabolism to replicate and form copies. These copies then break open the cell and spread to other cells. In this way, 'fragments of code may be transferred from the cells of one species to another, Man and Mouse, Monkey and Cat, by viruses or through other procedures'.[16] Here the organization of different forms of coding processes and their associated territories move in the direction of increasing deterritorialization. Deterritorialization is how territory gets invaded, relinquished or undone by means of decoding and transfer of materials that break it apart. The body gets disassembled by genetic transfer and disease into 'a number of more or less deterritorialized states'.[17] Here Deleuze and Guattari borrow the language of territorialization, deterritorialization, and reterritorialization from Paul Virilio to describe how the earth gets segmented and stratified by natural and human processes. In modern capitalism, the land and nonmodern societies get deterritorialized by military, financial and cultural means, and then they become reterritorialized under capitalism. In capitalism, deterritorialization and reterritorialization work together, but here Deleuze and Guattari attempt to think an absolute deterritorialization that would escape any and all reterritorialization.

Every deterritorialization is relative to its territory, and to its potential reterritorialization along different lines with different strata, forms, codings and expressions. At a certain point, however, deterritorialization can be associated with the plane or consistency, the body without organs, or the abstract machine as an absolute form of deterritorialization. 'In a certain sense,' they state, 'the acceleration of relative deterritorializations reaches the sound barrier,' and 'if they cross the barrier they reach the unformed, destratified element of the plane consistency.'[18] We have to be careful of this word acceleration, because absolute deterritorialization is not a giant accelerator, *pace* the bastardized Deleuzo-Guattarian movement that calls itself Accelerationism.[19] According to Deleuze and Guattari, 'what qualifies a deterritorialization is not its speed (some are very slow) but its nature'. Within every relative deterritorialization, there exists 'a perpetual immanence of absolute deterritorialization' with which it is related.[20]

There is an alignment of code or nucleic sequence that 'marks a threshold of deterritorialization', which gives it 'a new ability to be copied and makes the organism more deterritorialized than a crystal'. This nucleic sequence is contained with the state of the body in a way that allows it to both protect and reclaim its territory, and it exists in the form of the virus, which works as a sign to deterritorialize the body in a way that shows how absolute deterritorialization works. 'Only something deterritorialized is capable of reproducing itself,' but the virus gives us a glimpse of absolute deterritorialization in its line of flight *into* the body as a mad singularity and a free particle that disorders intensities.[21] We have to be careful; I am not advocating, promoting or celebrating the millions of deaths caused by the COVID-19 coronavirus, but rather attempting to read this pandemic as a sign of something that allows us to glimpse what Deleuze and Guattari call absolute deterritorialization, which is tremendously complicated and abstract.

Deleuze and Guattari are provocatively using machinic language, and they are also arguing that we need to comprehend the earth as not only a body without organs, or even a plane of consistency for all of the forms that are geologic, but more importantly as an abstract machine. The emergence of machines like computers and other processors of big data and powerful simulations allows us to see how the interactions among all of the strata (of the planet, of the body, of the socius...) in their interstitial assemblages, the – between B and A, enables the abstract machine to begin to 'unfold, to stand to full height, producing an illusion exceeding all strata, even though the machine itself belongs to a determinate stratum'.[22]

The machinic assemblages are distinct forms that are 'necessary for the relations between two strata to come about'.[23] These assemblages conjoin and detach; they constitute relations between and among phenomena that allow us to comprehend their interactions and organization. The problem is when we take these strata and their corresponding sedimentations for granted as causally conjoined in every natural or social assemblage. Assemblages are 'necessary for states of force and regimes of signs to intertwine their relations. Assemblages are necessary in order for the unity of compositions enveloped in a stratum, the relations between a given stratum and others, and the relation between these strata and the plane of consistency to be organized rather than random'.[24] These machinic assemblages produce the abstract machine that they presuppose, which develops along the plane of consistency, which is also a plane of immanence.

According to Deleuze and Guattari, a machinic assemblage is an interstratum because it 'regulates the relations between strata, as well as the relations between contents and expression on each stratum'. The machinic assemblage is also a metastratum because 'it is also in touch with the plane of consistency and effectuates the abstract machine'.[25] The combination of machinic assemblages and the abstract machines they generate can be described in terms of an overarching Mechanosphere.

Everything is part of the same Mechanosphere: there are no separate contents or stages, like a simple geological substratum, a living biosphere or a human social order. All of these phenomena intersect and interact in the most complex and disparate ways. The Mechanosphere gives us a name for the plane of consistency and all of its contents, but there is no higher or lower level, no hierarchy in the sense of a value judgement, no progression from less to more consciousness, morality or state of civilization that is explicit or implied in so many discussions of planetary evolution. Finally, there is the abolition of metaphor: 'All that consists is Real. There are electrons in person, veritable black holes, actual organites, authentic sign sequences. It's just that they have been uprooted from their strata, destratified, decoded, deterritorialized, and that is what makes their proximity and their interpenetration in the plane of consistency possible.'[26]

It's a question of how to think, how to even wrap our minds around what is occurring in such a staggering multiplicity of ways as we exceed the comfortable carrying capacity, resource availability and temperature levels *for us*. As we unleash new monstrosities, first of all the coronavirus that has brought large portions of the planet to a standstill, but also new forms of media streaming saturation, new and contested science – tele-technologies, nano-technologies, new and old financial and economic instruments of domination, new and absurd attempts to control and direct the war machine (Syria, Ukraine, Taiwan) and new forms of faith, fundamentalist, nihilistic, schizophrenic, progressive, illusory and even realistic.

The virus is a war machine

In their chapter of *A Thousand Plateaus* on Nomadology, Deleuze and Guattari explain that a war machine is irreducible to the State. The State exists as a stratum, and it is formed by the double articulation they analyse in their earlier chapter on 'The Geology of Morals'. The war machine, however, 'is not contained within this apparatus'. The war machine 'is of another species, another nature, another origin than the State apparatus'.[27] Deleuze and Guattari use examples from political and military history, but *here* the virus is a war machine and the body is a State, and this is not simply an analogy or metaphor because of the nature of the abstract machine and how it is encompassed by the plane of consistency, as quoted above. Deleuze and Guattari disentangle the war machine from the State, which means that 'the State has no war machine of its own'.[28] It has to appropriate and deploy a war machine from outside. The Body appropriates the immune system as its military to counter the original war machines of bacteria and viruses.

Furthermore, the existence of the war machine attests to an epistemology that opposes the royal science that serves the State to a 'nomad' or 'minor science' that adopts a more complex nonlinear model. The royal science of the State is Platonic-Aristotelian because it posits an overarching form that subjects and organizes matter, whereas nomad science attends more directly to material forces and their operations. A positive science of virology that treats the virus as an integral form in itself is a minor science as opposed to the royal science that only posits the virus as an enemy to be segregated or destroyed. Nomad science is prohibited by royal science, and this 'State science continually imposes its form of sovereignty on the inventions of nomad science'.[29] Here the sovereignty of the Body is maintained over against the minor agents of terror that infiltrate and subvert its organization.

Tiny agents are targeted for elimination by the sovereign State of the body and its universal logic. While the State assigns its subjects roles and function that they must obey, the nomadic war machine '*distributes people (or animals* [or bacteria, or viruses]) *in an open space*, one that is indefinite and noncommunicating'.[30] While the space assigned by the State is striated, nomadic space is smooth: 'the nomad distributes himself in a smooth space; he occupies, inhabits, holds that space'.[31] The virus operates in a smooth vector space, distributing itself across interstices between organisms, between strata, inserting itself inside the interior of the proper sovereign body.

We read Deleuze and Guattari and we think that they are celebrating violence and war; they are agents of destruction. However, this is extremely naïve, because '*the war machine does not necessarily have war as its object*'.[32] The war machine becomes war under specific conditions of opposition to and by the State apparatus that is set up to annihilate it. According to their analysis, 'war is neither the condition nor the object of the war machine, but necessarily accompanies or completes it; speaking like Derrida, we would say that war is the "supplement" of the war machine'.[33] War becomes inevitable whenever there is the refusal of the war machinic assemblage to be assimilated into the State apparatus. It is rather the State that '*appropriates* the war machine, subordinates it to its "political" *aims*, and gives it war as its direct *object*'.[34] This is the creation of a gigantomachy, a World War Machine in whose shadow we live and fight. The appropriation of the war machine by the State or the Body constitutes an immunological situation where the weapons of the war machine are unleashed against it in a cascade of annihilation.

This World War Machine has grown stronger and stronger during the twentieth century and into the twenty-first: 'We have seen it assign as its objective a peace still more terrifying than fascist death; we have seen it maintain or instigate the most terrible type of local wars as parts of itself; we have seen it set its sights on a new type of enemy, no longer another State, or even another regime, but the "unspecified enemy"'.[35] The

Unspecified Enemy is the terrorist, the activist, the insurgent, and alien, the social justice warrior who threatens the sovereign State apparatus and its functioning under capitalist neoliberalism. The key point here is that the war machine is not essentially related to a physical State of war; it possesses a variable relation to war itself.

At the end of the chapter, Deleuze and Guattari reflect on the fact that they tried to 'assign the invention of the war machine to the nomads' but this is not possible. 'It is not the nomad who defines this constellation of characteristics' that constitutes the war machine; 'it is this constellation that defines the nomad, and at the same time the essence of the war machine.'[36] It is not the nomadic virus that constitutes the war machine, but rather the constellation of a smooth space of displacement, a creative line of flight, and a plane of consistency that creates both the virus as nomadic agent *and* the war machine that it delivers to the Body. War machines can make war '*only on condition that they simultaneously create something else*, if only new nonorganic social relations'.[37] These new nonorganic social relations that result from the war of the coronavirus on humanity attest to a power of deterritorialization, an absolute deterritorialization of the earth, whose forces 'live and blaze their way for a new earth'.[38]

A new nomos of the earth

In the Conclusion of *A Thousand Plateaus*, Deleuze and Guattari return to the question of absolute deterritorialization that they raised earlier in 'The Geology of Morals'. Here they identify absolute deterritorialization with the earth; 'the earth, the glacial, is Deterriorialization par excellence: that is why it belongs to the Cosmos, and presents itself as the material through which human beings tap into cosmic forces'. In this way, Deterritorialization 'can be called the creator of the earth – of a new land, a universe, not just a reterritorialization'.[39] What does this mean? The movements of relative deterritorialization and reterritorialization take place on the same earth, or the same global plane, whereas the absolute deterritorialization that is associated here with the earth creates a new earth, a new nomos of earth that is 'qualitatively different from relative movement' upon the same planet.[40]

Absolute deterritorialization opens up a new vision of earth by means of a complex of totally different lines of flight. Deterritorialization is absolute when 'it brings about the creation of a new earth, in other words, when it connects lines of flight, raises them to the power of an abstract line, or draws a plane of consistency'.[41] This abstract vital line of flight seeks a new, smooth perspective from which to think and develop an entirely new plane of consistency, and the virus is an agent that helps accomplish this work. Relative deterritorialization is the globe of capitalism; 'the earth girded, encompassed, overcoded, conjugated as the subject of a mortuary and suicidal organization surrounding it on all sides'. This contrasts with absolute deterritorialization, which lies deep within relative deterritorialization, and comprehends 'the earth consolidated, connected with the Cosmos, brought into the Cosmos following lines of creation that cut across it as so many becomings'.[42]

Global capitalism has overcoded, subjugated and stratified the earth and all of its inhabitants. We desperately need new lines of flight into the smooth spaces vital for creation and destratification. We need to subtract ourselves from these exhausted reterritorializations of the same territory. We need to find the limit and one of the vectors to this point comes from following the line of flight of the virus as it cuts across bodies, organs, milieus and hemispheres, replicating itself in a mad operation of differentiation. This does not mean that we celebrate the death that the virus has caused; it means that we open ourselves up to thinking like a virus beyond the limits of corporate capitalist control.

The absolute deterritorialization the virus implies suggests that we think across species to create entirely New Solidarities that stretch and burst our conceptions of kin. We are embedded in too many entanglements with other non-human organisms to survive alone. We must rethink what it means to be in community, and take on the task of making kin beyond any form of familial kinship. This is what Donna Haraway advocates in her book *Staying with the Trouble*. She says that 'the task is to make kin in lives of inventive connection as a practice of learning to live and die well with each other in a thick present'.[43] Rather than an Anthropocene or a Capitalocene, Haraway suggests that we are living in the Chthulucene, a name that indicates a thick presence for earth-beings. Chthulucene names 'a kind of timeplace for learning to stay with the trouble of living and dying in response-ability on a damaged earth'.[44] This Chthulucene is a name that resonates with Deleuze and Guattari's conception of a new earth.

We need to think and comprehend the pandemic more rhizomatically, to see how the spread of the virus consists in not only a devastating illness but also a nomadic war machine that is deterritorializing the globe, creating new assemblages, alliances and pandemic solidarities. Here we can think about the text on *Pandemic Solidarity: Mutual Aid During the COVID-19 Crisis*, produced by the ensemble Colectiva Sembrar. This book connects mutual aid movements around the world in their struggle to practise care for the vulnerable and their efforts to envision a humane life beyond the devastation of neoliberal capitalism. As Rebecca Solnit explains, the two most important lessons are: one, that people already 'knew how to self-organize, and that horizontal, democratic means were what worked, over and over, in place after place', and the other is 'the joy they seemed to find, even in the worst of circumstances, in finding the agency to act, and the communion of acting together'.[45] This important analysis needs to be expanded beyond its stereotypical humanism as new solidarities are formed among and across species and other forms, while a desperate neoliberalism denies its functioning and clings to outmoded and outstripped modes of globalism.

In a short response to the COVID-19 situation, Catherine Malabou suggests that the only way to truly liberate oneself from the confinement and isolation inflicted by the pandemic is to find deeper space of confinement within confinement. 'I noticed that writing only became possible,' she reflects, 'when I reached such a confinement within confinement, a place in the place where nobody could enter and that at the same time was the condition for my exchanges with others.'[46] I am suggesting that this is a truly creative space because it corresponds to the smooth space of absolute deterritorialization that Deleuze and Guattari help us conceive. We need to find an absolute deterritorialization within relative movements of deterritorialization and reterritorialization. We need to not simply deplore and despise the effects of the virus; we also need to think like a virus, to follow it on its line of flight deeper within us than our skin and our organs. We need to find that space of absolute confinement that is the place of genuine revolutionary care and liberation, from which we reach out to embrace new and entirely nomadic forms of solidarity.

Notes

1 John M. Barry, *The Great Influenza: The Story of the Deadliest Pandemic in History* (New York: Penguin Books, 2004), p. 248.
2 Ibid., pp. 249–250.
3 See 'Covid-19 and the Flu', *American Society for Microbiology*, 7 October 2021: https://asm.org/Articles/2020/July/COVID-19-and-the-Flu
4 Gilles Deleuze, *Difference and Repetition*, trans. Paul Patton (New York: Columbia University Press, 1994), p. 224.
5 See https://www.cdc.gov/flu/pandemic-resources/1918-commemoration/1918-pandemic-history.htm
6 Jacques Derrida, 'Faith and Knowledge: The Two Sources of "Religion" at the Limits of Reason Alone', in *Religion*, eds. Jacques Derrida and Gianni Vattimo (Stanford: Stanford University Press, 1998), p. 51.
7 See Giovanni Borradori, *Philosophy in a Time of Terror: Dialogues with Jürgen Habermas and Jacques Derrida* (Chicago: University of Chicago Press, 2003), pp. 101.
8 Ibid., p. 102.
9 See Gilles Deleuze, 'Postscript on the Societies of Control', *OCTOBER*, Vol. 59, The MIT Press, 1992, pp. 3–7.
10 Gilles Deleuze and Félix Guattari, *A Thousand Plateaus: Capitalism and Schizophrenia*, trans. Brian Massumi (Minneapolis: University of Minnesota Press, 1987), p. 10.
11 Ibid., p. 10.
12 Ibid., p. 11.
13 Ibid. p. 40.
14 Ibid., p. 40.
15 Ibid., p. 53.
16 Ibid., p. 53.
17 Ibid., p. 53.
18 Ibid., p. 56.
19 See *#Accelerate: The Accelerationist Reader*, ed. Robin Mackay and Armin Avanessian (London: Urbanomic, 2014).
20 Deleuze and Guattari, *A Thousand Plateaus*, p. 56.
21 Ibid. pp. 59–60.
22 Ibid., p. 63.
23 Ibid., p. 71.
24 Ibid., p. 71.
25 Ibid., p. 73.
26 Ibid., p. 69.
27 Ibid., p. 352.
28 Ibid., p. 355.
29 Ibid., p. 362.
30 Ibid., p. 380 (emphasis in original).
31 Ibid., p. 381.

32 Ibid., p. 416 (emphasis in original).
33 Ibid., p. 417.
34 Ibid., p. 420.
35 Ibid., p. 422.
36 Ibid., p. 423.
37 Ibid., p. 423 (emphasis in original).
38 Ibid., p. 423.
39 Ibid., p. 509.
40 Ibid., p. 509.
41 Ibid., p. 510.
42 Ibid., p. 510.
43 Donna J. Haraway, *Staying with the Trouble: Making Kin in the Chthulucene* (Durham: Duke University Press, 2016), p. 1.
44 Ibid., p. 2.
45 *Pandemic Solidarity: Mutual Aid During the COVID-19 Crisis*, ed. Maria Sitrin and the Colectiva Sembrar (London: Pluto Press, 2020), p. xiii.
46 Catherine Malabou, 'To Quarantine from Quarantine: Rousseau, Robinson Crusoe, and "I"', In the Moment, *Critical Inquiry* Blog, 23 March 2020. https://critinq.wordpress.com/2020/03/23/to-quarantine-from-quarantine-rousseau-robinson-crusoe-and-i/

References

Barry, J. M. (2004), *The Great Influenza*. New York: Penguin.

Borradori, G. (2003), *Philosophy in a Time of Terror: Dialogues with Jürgen Habermas and Jacques Derrida*. Chicago: University of Chicago Press.

Centers for Disease Control and Prevention. (2018, 21 March), *History of 1918 Flu Pandemic*. Centers for Disease Control and Prevention. Retrieved 4 September 2022, from https://www.cdc.gov/flu/pandemic-resources/1918-commemoration/1918-pandemic-history.htm

Deleuze, G. (1992), Postscript on the Societies of Control. *October*, *59*, 3–7. http://www.jstor.org/stable/778828

Deleuze, G. (1994), *Difference and Repetition* (P. Patton, Trans.). New York: Columbia University Press.

Deleuze, G., and Guattari, F. (1987), *A Thousand Plateaus: Capitalism and Schizophrenia* (B. Massumi, Trans.). Minneapolis: University of Minnesota Press.

Derrida, J., and Vattimo, G. (1998), Faith and Knowledge: The Two Sources of 'Religion' at the Limits of Reason Alone. In J. Derrida (Ed.), *Religion* (p. 51). Essay, Stanford: Stanford University Press.

Hagen, A. (2020, 31 July), *Covid-19 and the Flu*. ASM.org. Retrieved 4 September 2022, from https://asm.org/Articles/2020/July/COVID-19-and-the-Flu

Haraway, D. J. (2016), *Staying with the Trouble: Making Kin in the Chthulucene*. Durham: Duke University Press.

Mackay, R., and Avanessian, A. (Eds.). (2014), *#Accelerate: The Accelerationist Reader*. London: Urbanomic.

Malabou, C. (2021), To quarantine from quarantine: Rousseau, Robinson Crusoe, and 'I'. *Critical Inquiry*, *47*(S2). https://doi.org/10.1086/711426

Sitrin, M., and Sembrar, C. (2020), *Pandemic Solidarity: Mutual Aid During the Covid-19 Crisis*. London: Pluto Press.

2

Beyond Control: Technology, Post-Faciality and the Dance of the Abstract

Brad Evans and Chantal Meza

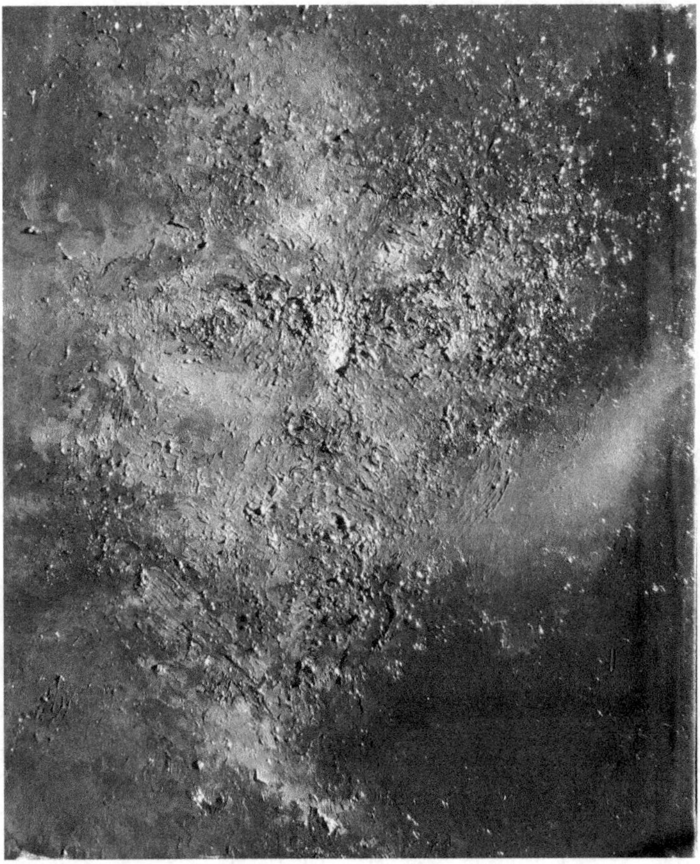

Figure 2.1 Artwork: Chantal Meza, Self Portrait, 2021. Oil on canvas, 55 × 66 cm. © Chantal Meza.

The Nomad doesn't physically move. Theirs is more an ontological positioning vis-à-vis the sedentary ambitions of the State and its captive political formations. Rather than moving across physical space, nomadism then is the liberation of thought from all forms of capture and containment. Or at least this was the theory of *Nomadology* proposed by Gilles Deleuze and Felix Guattari.[1] But what does this conception of the nomad as being the one who stays yet freely wanders mean in this post-pandemic world? Is such an account of becoming not fully in keeping with the logics of power, which have turned every thought into an algorithmic opportunity to learn more about the self, every single body into a surveillance concern, every home into a veritable border, and every street into a hostile terrain that is to be mapped in advance? A logic that insists humanity will only find its freedom in and through digital technologies, which have been also fully embraced by the post-liberal left? Whatever one thinks of the need for the lockdown and the new bio-political demands to vaccinate the entire planet, it's clear the crisis has ushered in a moment in which the power of technology and its reach have increased exponentially. Unrivalled in fact in its ability to transform the lived conditions on earth, while ushering in a new sacred paradigm as the technological embrace is presented to us as the only means for saving an endangered humanity from itself, this new architecture for power is what we have elected to call the global techno-theodicy.[2]

Deleuze partly anticipated this condition in his short influential essay 'Postscript on Control Societies'.[3] Yet what's also most immediately apparent with this essay is the way he focuses more on the *physical* movement of bodies, and how such movements may be tracked and opened to new kinds of interventions. The onset of Control Societies thus begins by proposing a new understanding on the body's relationship to movement and its continuous assay in mutable locations across space and time. It is all about critiquing the organization of power and the replacement of one kind of society – *sovereign societies*, with another – *societies of control*. Witnessing the 'general breakdown of all sites of confinement', for Deleuze older linear models were being replaced by a general surveillance of the species that is all about 'coexisting metastable states of a single modulation, a sort of universal transmutation'. What makes this all possible, he contends, is a shift away from an *analogue* condition in which variables, despite their disciplinary subjugation, retained a certain independence and distinct positioning, towards the language of the *digital* made possible by the revolutions in 'cybernetic machinery', 'information technology' and 'instantaneous communication'. In short, it was a new organization for power that was fully capable of absorbing nomadic tendencies and the desire to break free from the disciplinary confines of the analogue world.

None of this reads as controversial today. The mantra that 'information is power' is repeated to the point of monotony. That the digital network has become the social morphology for the age,[4] redefining all social relations is not in doubt. While this 'advancement' has radically altered all aspects of planetary life, it has also led to a notable updating of Deleuze's provocation considering the changing architectures for power. This has included addressing the global ambitions of capitalism and the importance of foregrounding networks in terms of conceptualizing the operations of power and the organization of resistance;[5] reassessing the role borders play in the control of movements;[6] along with showing how late liberal security regimes were underwritten by the language of complexity, emergence and the network form.[7] While this has also led to a reconceptualization of bio-politics as understood to be primarily concerned with the control of circulations and what this means for the securitization of peoples, it would in turn provoke a rethink on the logic of violence in even more vital ways than originally conceptualized by both Foucault and later Deleuze. As Jean Baudrillard observed:

> The violence of networks and the virtual is viral: it is the violence of benign extermination, operating at the genetic communicational level; a violence of consensus. . . . A viral violence in the sense that it does not operate head-on, but by contiguity, contagion, and chain reaction, its aim being the loss of all our immunities. And also in the sense that, contrary to the historical violence of negation, this virus operates hyper-positively, like cancerous cells, through endless proliferation, excrescence, and metastasis. Between virtuality and virality, there is a kind of complicity.[8]

Like his previous concerns with nomadism against the state, Deleuze was also acutely aware that the advent of Control Societies would have a marked impact on how we come to imagine and produce subjects. With education being central to the active creation of subjectivities through process of continuous intervention, so we would encounter the rise of the 'digital individual' or what is noted in the text to be 'dividuals'. These new subjects are both seduced by a certain idea of immanence, and yet would nevertheless increasingly find that virtual borders existed everywhere. Now, there is no need to rehearse here the earlier debates on whether Deleuze's ontology and its concern with becoming was fully in keeping with the logics of late capitalism.[9] As argued elsewhere, the concept of complexity and emergence promoted by bourgeoise liberals was far removed from the liberated idea of becoming Deleuze had in mind.[10] Nor are we concerned whether Deleuze's theorization on Control Societies has been proven right. That seems self-evident. What concerns us is how Deleuze's theory no longer goes far enough in this post-pandemic world. It demands rethinking, for while earlier critiques of Control Societies were pushed by radical thinkers who were very much concerned with the technologization of life and how this could be complemented by the selective imposition of borders – ones that were porous enough to allow certain forms of circulation and yet fully prohibitive to others, what we have seen in the past few years is how critique has turned into both acceptance and promotion. Many on the so-called illiberal left have in fact been the most vociferous advocates of hyper-technologization, while insisting that the State enforces the widespread conditions of containment and surveillance.

But this is not simply about learning to live with the virus. What's been taking place is a profound acceleration in the technologization of life, which makes Deleuze's theory seem rather primitive by comparison. We are, in short, in a condition today that is truly *Beyond Control* as the triumph of the technical imagination is writ large as it seeks to colonize every creative expression, every thought, every projection, every concern; making a nomadism of technological abstraction fully possible, while denying the human any autonomy to freely roam or to even imagine some viable escape (especially intellectual). Indeed, if we can accept that power has become attuned to the logic of nomadism, actively encouraging us to wander amongst virtual terrains in the seduced comforts of our own homes in which heightened bio-political surveillance has become so routine we actively participate in its welcoming, what's needed is to both update and depart from Deleuze's important critique. This requires us to contend with what might this vision of a Control Society mean in relation to a post-liberal bio-politics? A time which has demanded an open and allegiant fall back into forms of containment (house, school, workplace, village, province, Nation), while fully collapsing the species into the technological. To partly counter this in the limited space remaining, we will now focus on two other issues that concerned Deleuze. Namely, to focus on the relationship between faciality and imperceptibility as this relates to the remarkable onset and radical support given to the covering of one's face in the name of a post-liberal bio-politics – one that placed humanity central to its claims, along with a return to the question of movement through the abstract line and what this might mean for resistance in an age of unrivalled technological power.

Observed from a distance, one of the most remarkable things to witness about the early stages of the global pandemic was the ease at which governments could tolerate their citizens covering most of their faces.[11] This would have seemed inconceivable only a few years prior, as liberal states in particular were investing millions in facial recognition systems to combat the threats posed by Islamic fundamentalists. Terror would thus become a condition of possibility for heightened and lasting security measures, which in turn would be rolled out to wider populations. We have known that faciality is integral to notions of identity. This seems particularly acute in Western societies where the face is the loci for one's individuality, and by that very token their sense of expressive freedom. The reason why beheading, for example, is seen as so intolerable for those in the West can reasonably be explained in terms of its ontological significance, the severing of the subject of their very subjectiveness.[12] But such faciality has also been the focus of critique. Most notably by Deleuze and Guattari, who understood how faciality was integral to the formation of master signifiers and the representational model for power. As they wrote in *A Thousand Plateaus*:

> Faces are not basically individual; they define zones of frequency and probability, delimit a field that neutralises in advance any expressions or connections unamenable to the appropriate significations. Similarly, the form of subjectivity, whether consciousness or passion, would remain absolutely empty if faces did not form a loci of resonance that select the sensed or mental reality and make it conform in advance to a dominant reality. . . . The face constructs the wall of the signifier, the frame or screen. The face digs the hole that subjectification needs in order to break through; it constitutes the black hole of subjectivity as consciousness or passion, the camera, the third eye.[13]

To 'dismantle the face', Deleuze and Guattari would find a meaningful escape thorough the desire to *become-imperceptible*. 'Movement has an essential relation to the imperceptible,' they write, 'it is by nature imperceptible.'[14] But what does this mean in a time when movement is so colonized and tracked that it can be immanently co-opted and turned back upon itself? And what becomes of the secret when power ethically demands that every feeling be spoken? A revealing that's also of course fully in keeping with the affective turn in technologization. There is still no doubt a great appeal to imperceptibility, especially as all forms of rights to privacy are being openly destroyed. We need to deny the machine full knowledge, as much as we need to retain what it means to be human in the twenty-first century. Related to this, we find much to agree with in Deleuze and Guattari's disruption of the representational model for the human, from the intimate engagements with the violence of Francis Bacon, onto the wider ideas of becoming-animal, which breaks open the imitative and mimetic theory of art. And yet something has been lost here in translation, both in terms of how the notion of becoming has made the human appear more and more vulnerable on account of some claimed ecological universalism, along with how claims of being post-human have collapsed the human fully into a technological paradigm. Becoming imperceptible should not mean that we lose the exceptionalism of the human condition. Humans are exceptional. That does not mean they are naturally top of the food chain. Nor does it mean they occupy the centre of the universe, thereby authoring hierarchies in their name. The exceptional is not a relationship of hierarchy at all. It belongs to the outside. It retains its uniqueness. Yes, it is prone to adaptation and change. And yes, it can mutate, while being penetrated and host to other life forms as the body reveals an ecology of the self. But the denial of the human is a denial of its existence. It is a denial in short of its own singular creation.

Returning to the black hole of subjectivity, we would like to move this around or at least be more determined in our assumptions. *Ontology is a void.*[15] It is a black hole. A site of pure potentiality. Now of course there is a marked difference here between ontology and faciality as much as there is a marked difference between ontology and subjectivity. But what really concerns us is the reason why faciality no longer matters. And what does this mean for the battle over the meaning of the abstract, which for Deleuze and Guattari is key to understanding the political stakes? If 'The face is politics' after all, as the authors have rightly contended, this is wholly dependent on the creation of an *abstract machine of faciality*, which is technically committed to its *over-coding*. Of course, it is true that in the contemporary moment there is still considerable interest in the complex mapping of faces, especially its racialization.[16] This means there is a need to still be alert to the racial biases of technology, notably how the algorithmic coding points to inbuilt forms of prejudice that are part of the technological design. But such concerns are only part of a wider story, which is more committed to the annihilation of the human. The pandemic showed this. Some may invariably counter that masks were only a temporary measure, and besides, most people had to be off the streets anyway. Our reading is different. Faces no longer matter and the mask conceals nothing of real value. The face has become disposable as true as the image of its all too fleeting appearance and consumption. Dominant forms of power no longer need the face as such to create a locus of resonance. Faces can be duplicated. They can be simulated. They can be warped. They can be artificially created. Indeed, as the pandemic showed, the face is now rather incidental when it comes to knowing, tracking and colonizing life. Faces in fact, we might say, suffer from being too bio-political! They are too material; they rot before our very eyes. They are a constant reminder of our mortal finitude. Faces are death masks, projecting with each passing second a singular future that's already being undone. No longer perfect, we now see them as Francis Bacon intended, screaming silently at the world. Too limiting, too overlaid with testimony to the marks of a life (which the technology encourages us to erase as part of its attempt to open a deeper entry), faces have too much autonomy, still retaining a capacity to hide things, to keep secrets. That is why so much effort today goes into having us believe in the fallibility of being human.[17] We should no longer trust our bodies, no longer believe in what the face has to say, no longer, as Paul Virilio noted, believe our eyes.[18] Technological power has a different referent in mind – the life of the mind. Sure, it is a power that still invokes the bio-political, the vulnerability of bodies, to justify unrivalled access into the depths of the body as a complex dataset. But the bio-political is merely the point of entry into a much deeper concern with the neuropolitical. This is why contemporary debates about inserting micro-chips into the brain for the purposes of health (notably dementia and autism) are not incidental. The mind has become the territory. And the ambition is precisely to conquer its creativity; to render all known secrets apparent, which in turn means fully over-coding the poetic abstract was a technical vision of neurological becoming.[19] This raises a crucial question. What happens to the idea of becoming imperceptible when power no longer needs faciality to author its control over the human form? What in other words remains of imperceptibility if the neuro-political power of technology has already entered those uncharted black holes wherein our most intimate, creative and guarded secrets were kept? Or to put it in even more critical terms, can we not imagine a notion of the secret that belongs to the poetic abstract but has nothing to do with the 'war machine'?[20]

Might we not be accused of falling back into a certain technological determinism here? The idea that technology has been the motor of history was well made during the twentieth century. Arguably the most celebrated and notable in this regard was Marshall McLuhan whose many books would foreground the problem of technology, especially its violence and depoliticizations, in important ways.[21] Others however were less convinced, none more so that Raymond Williams who insisted upon a more social reading of technology and its impact on society. While this was alluded to in his now classical text *Modern Tragedy*,[22] it would become more explicit in a chapter titled 'The Technology and the Society' in *Television: Technology and Cultural Form*.[23] Working against the perceived techno-determinism of McLuhan, Williams insisted upon the prevalence of social over technological in the formation of human processes. 'Determination is a real social process,' Williams wrote, 'but never (as in some theological and some Marxist versions) . . . a wholly controlling, wholly predicting set of causes. On the contrary, the reality of determination is the setting of limits and the exertion of pressures, within which variable social practices are profoundly affected but never necessarily controlled.'[24] This approach would be later developed by Deleuze and Guattari, who also insisted that 'the machine' was always socially conceived before it was technological. Or to put it another way, society will produce the technologies it desires (even if such desires end up being the source of our oppression). But what happens when desire desires its own determinacy? What happens when the social is willingly abdicated and given fully over to machines that promise to rid us of our own fallibilities? What happens when the machine is programmed to be more epistemically and even linguistically astute? What happens when we therefore desire our own technological extinction as though it were a human liberation? This is the state we live in today. A threshold has been crossed, as the technological now shapes the social, feeding off the desired inadequacies of humans, paraded as a means through which the concept of humanity may finally be revealed, while parasitic to the affective currencies of the affected who broadcast the need for something to save them from their own excessiveness. Industrial determinacy was powered by raw human energy, which still made man a master of his own technological devising as his ambitions for worldly conquest and inevitable machinic destruction ruled the earth. Digital determinacy has replaced the social logics of the old with a new nervous vitalism, which now looks upon every ontological claim the human possessed as primordial by comparison. This is not the Newtonian determinism critiqued by Williams. It's a technological vision of species life that demands full immersion, and within which the social is but a necessary fragile component.

The desire to socially give oneself over to the power of 'intelligent machines' has been exemplified by Paul Dicken, who imagines an artificial world where life now needs a adapt to the wider technological conditions for rule. Foregrounding his concern with 'semantic content', this is a vision in which everything is reduced to a competition over the power of the technical imagination (a competition humans are fated to lose as they simply don't have the grammatical fortitude to compare), and where the only capacity for excessiveness – the only abstract, is the sole preserve of technology. This posits a post-philosophical future wherein the human is truly seconded, if not rendered altogether redundant as far as creative thought is concerned. Post-humanist assumptions thus inevitably return here as thought might be presented as a mere facilitator for survival. Whatever happened to the poetic and the human abstract is fully written out of this technical script. As he writes:

> [Alan] Turing wondered what it would take for us to treat a machine as if it were talking. The resulting history of the Turing Test has largely been an exercise more in human foible than machine intelligence; Joseph Weizenbaum's early successes with ELIZA simply involved aping the psychoanalytic technique of turning every statement into a question, and when in doubt, asking its interlocutor about their mother. But perhaps Turing was looking at it the wrong way round. As we learn to manage our expectations in conformity with algorithmic decisions, modify our inputs to machine-friendly format, and slowly abandon any pretense at nuance in the quick-fire forum of social media – communication without conversation – it begins to look as if it might be easier to build a human that can talk to a computer, rather than the other way around. Then the important philosophical question will be if we have anything interesting left to say.[25]

We are acutely aware here of how our analysis might be taken as another duplicitous way of suggesting we live in a post-racial moment. We are making no such claim. The legacy of colonization still bleeds deep and its micro-segmentary divisions are all too apparent in this lock-down world. What we are however also saying is that coloniality has moved it, and like its earlier variants it is able to absorb bodies and minds regardless of colour. Moreover, within this colonial model, identity matters for identity as an immanently commodifiable fashion is what drives on the 'political' need for continued and more pronounced technological advancement. Deleuze once infamously declared: 'If you are trapped in the dream of the other, you are fucked.' How little we seem to have learned as we continue to speak on behalf of others, partly fucked by their good intentions and royally fucked by the new systems they throw us into. Still doubling sameness, how the self-resemblance of being reappears intrinsic to identity. The idea that the dominant order for power still centres on the aged white man makes no sense to us. The master signifier of today has no signification. It is as ephemeral as the digital cloud from which it emerges and draws all things in. In Bryan Singer's classic *The Usual Suspects*, Keyser Söze mischievously remarked that 'The greatest trick the devil ever pulled was convincing the world he did not exist.' Our wager is that the greatest trick the devil has come to play was to convince the world he was God and that some old demon remained the devil.

If we wanted to be as crude as the technocrats of reason, we could suggest that their world is measured by *length and duration*. Armed with their own progressive faith, the future is a problem which ultimately needs to be prolonged as long as possible. The artist, poet and critical philosopher have a different vision in mind that is measured more by the *depths of existence*. If the technocrat thus seeks to ward off the void for as long as possible, even if that means suspending life in some catatonic state, just for the sake of confirming the sacredness of its appearance, the poetic sensibility strives instead to befriend the void as they know its ontological reckoning. But the social and human death of the technologist is all too apparent. They would rather cut off their arm and replace it with an artificial one if it meant they could perfectly mimic the style of a Picasso. They would replace their veins full of blood with a digital nervous system if it meant their age could be doubled. They would willingly open the mind to a colonial implant if it meant preserving their everlasting thoughts. And they would replace their mortal bodies altogether with a virtual soul if it led to the promise of an eternal life. Theirs is a dream of a conflict-free existence, yet as neurotic as the birds in Klee's composition. Indeed, the technological mind works to actualize and amplify the neurotic state; marked by a dream for everlasting life that is haunted by the presence of a void which cannot be eliminated. For were it to do so, the technologist learns, one ultimately obliterates the human and the ontology of the self. That is why technology will never 'save us' despite its sacred claims. On the contrary, it forces us to endure, to life immersed within an accelerating state of technical and calculated becoming. And that is why the current return on the left to 'progressivism' reveals how its radicalism has also been fully absorbed and its desires appropriated. Having given themselves over to a technological dream, the radical progressive is fully in keeping with the sacred demands of the global techno-theodicy, which no longer need Prometheus, but the flat and vulnerable resilient life that has already created a simulacrum of the fire. Hence claiming to foresee everything; what they really see are mere fragments of nothing at all.

Art becomes our counter here as we imagine a world that doesn't abdicate what it means to be human.[26] The canvas appears as a white screen. Is this whiteness not also a void as indicated by Malevich? Or is it a wall that is as impenetrable as it is violently set and so rationally determined in advance for us? Before the potential composition is even encountered, there is the ritual. The mixing of the colours, the cutting of the knife into the pigments that bleeds anew like a piece of unidentified meat on a butcher's block. This is done is silence, except for the orchestral music playing in the background. The cutting of the knife works in harmony with the slow movement of the violinists bow, both of which remind us that even before anything happens, the artist, the painter, the musician, each is compelled by the intention of the poetic gesture, which makes the instrument always secondary. Art requires its atmosphere, the becoming music of the paint, the becoming ambient of the impenetrable white, the becoming intense of the artist who is yet to paint a single stroke. But the artist soon becomes this atmosphere. The palm of the hands starts to emit with the sweat of anticipation, they punch the canvas to let it know that the presence of the artist can no longer be denied. She is here. She is the brush, she is the paint, she is the canvas the moment the touch turns into the appearance of that first line. But there's a further becoming that's more complex. A digital screen reflects nothing. The artist knows this. Yet as she gazes into the mirror on the wall besides that offers back a reflection of herself, moving as with life into its deep halls of memory, distorting her own very image before her eyes as she tries to paint what she immanently sees, so the canvas too becomes a mirror, but of a different order of reflection. This is not about doubling. The artist is now triangulated – the self, the mirror and the canvas. A fated triangle perhaps between perpetrator, victim and witness? Or maybe human, existence and the void? There is no mimesis taking place here. Why would the artist want to mimic themselves anyway? Nor is this a confession, let alone an attempt to reveal the person she only wished the world to know. The artist is entering into a becoming with a reflection of herself so that she may become anew. Yes, she has her tools and her techniques. But these are never defining and never mastering.

Slowly the blacks and purples reveal themselves through the artist's delicate rotations that speak to styles that have been visually echoed across the sands of time. And let us not forget, the echo too is never a copy of the original. It works to its own unique sound and rhythm in its own space and in its own projected time. Does it ever really stop? Maybe we just don't know how to listen? Back to the composition, the outline of a head gradually appears; the artist gently guides the brush as a lover would caress a face. She knows these lines intimately, yet still she seems uncertain. Who really is the girl in the mirror? Is she not a stranger who has now finally appeared on the horizon of today? The strokes soon become more determined, more tremendous, more confident about the disfigurements she wilfully authors. And, yet, still, the tenderness remains. There's still a slowness to the work. The purples reflect the ambient light, and the faint stroke lines of the brush could be mistaken for the beautiful hair of the artist herself. Everything is worked here in circles. Circles of light, circles of sound, circles of deformation. Some vortexes it seems can appear before us barely moving. Is gravity capable of explaining this? Or maybe the poetic has a different gravitational pull?

The artist takes a deep breath. She hesitates. The music is silent. Everything is possible. The silence reveals nothing. But it is everything. For within those secrets resides something truly untouchable – a true ontological void, that will forever remain the sole possession of the artist. This is only the beginning. A lighter shade of purple is applied. This adds depth to the first layering. The darkness rises. Her face is already several. It's more than just angles of vision. It's more than lines of perception. The contorted intimacy is a dance that is as sensual as a pack of wolves. And what of this face? In the most violent of strokes, the artist paints over the white space that was left for the eyes. Who is seeing here anyway? Does she see the mirror or the canvas? Or does the mirror look back? And what does the canvas see? Does the eye need to be so located anyway? Have we lost the capacity to see what is before us? She turns to the throat. The brush caresses again but could so easily be mistaken for a knife gliding across the neck as if to acknowledge that she is severing herself from herself. Yet still she breathes; all three of her. The self-portrait is now a layered form, as layered as the history being composed in this moment of reckoning. This is a world away from the artificial world of pixels. Nothing here is programmed in advance. Nothing enabled because of intelligent machinic design. Such complexity is resolutely human, even as the artist becomes the animal she always was. And yet it is a mistake to reduce this to a naturalism of a special kind. The face is as angelic as it is daemonic. It is as captivating as it is repulsive. It is as tender as it is brutal. It is as ancestral as it belongs to this present moment. Its purple is as red as it is black. A silhouette of depth.

The more the paint is applied, the more the canvas reflects too. Is the artist now looking at her reflection in the oil and simply looking into the mirror on the wall for some kind of confirmation? The oil certainly brings the ecology of the work to life, secreting a wetness that is as seductive as blood. A mouth and tongue briefly come into focus. It's as if the painting is gasping for air, yet thankful to be part of this disappearing existence. Only to vanish again. She has already painted herself a thousand times now. Fuck authentication. Fuck those eyes. Fuck that mouth. At least that's how the misjudged might read her intentions. But everything is as it's meant to be here. There are no mistakes to rectify. Just new lines of creation, different movements in light, alternative dances with the sound. The artist is now fully lost in the rhythms of the work, spending considerable time remixing the paint on the glass board, barely breathing herself, letting the work breathe for her. She sighs. It's a sign. It's still only the beginning. She sighs again. The dark red makes its appearance. The colour demands her respect. It has been so abused in the past. And yet also used in such exceptional ways. Does she feel the weight of the colour here more than her actual self-portrait? It seems that way. The lines and circles are less numerous now. Yet, as with life, sometimes less reveals more. Sometimes very little, almost nothing, means a great deal to those whose respect is already there. But upon reflection it seems this red is far from violent or abysmal. It's vital. It is what characterizes as the purple starts to fade and dry into the background dusk. Why does the face horrify us so? And why is so much blood spilled because we can't abide its bloodied presence? Surely no machine could capture this. It could learn the lines. It could recite Benjamin. But it will never bleed such poetic blood, never know the tender beauty of these red marks that are more than mere wounds or technical cuts that just might tell us something more about the artist's desires.

The artist stands bleeding. A brighter red appears. Is this really how she pictures herself? Yes. A thousand more times disturbed. But she doesn't see herself as some kind of martyr. There's no poetic heroism here. She merely is. And that's more than enough.

Yet she still wants more. More layering, more depth, more to a life that cannot be flattened by some technical miracle or happenstance. What might a technician have to say about this anyway? They may retrace the lines, analyse the pigments, reveal back the exact way it was painted, and even which line came first. None of which would reveal anything. Without its atmosphere and unknown intentions, the painting is but a technical puzzle, which is a nothing of the worst possible kind. A nothing as trivial as it is banal. But the artist has already dismissed such an account of her life and returns to the red. It darkens on the canvas. Time weighs, but not always for the worse. Nobody is alone in the company of this colour. She is not merely projecting a vitalism. Its abstract becoming projects its own vitalism, which forces the artist to take breath at the sight of its immersions. If there is a beauty here, it's not on the surface of anything. The wrath of beauty has always been an artificially constructed affair. That's why poetics is no mere artifice. It is only artifactually construed by the technocratic mind. Absently apparent. Beauty is as deep as the blackened purples that are now only barely visible. And beauty is as rich as the regal reds, which deepen the appearance of this life in all its voiding.

The movements now become more strident. The canvas needs to be filled. Faces can too easily look like faces on the face of things. To become a face that's imperceptible to the facilizing gods of the old and the technically effacing gods of the new has become the challenge for these purifying times. Are we even looking upon the face at all? Or maybe we are now seeing the face from within? Seeing a more intimate reflection of the self that only the artist is able to see and chooses to give but a glimpse? To become a face that has such depth means to undo the privilege afforded to all known surfaces. It is to gaze upon from within, to feel the immersion of the face of the stranger who will never be fully encountered. It is to properly abstract the face so that it may be reimagined anew. It is a gaze upon the face that is as free as the air and as swirling as the vortex of time. It is to come face to face with something that cannot be explained by whatever intelligent machine we care to devise, cannot be understood in whatever posthumanism guise, yet cannot be shown to be false all the same. Becoming such a face is to have no recognition, other than to be recognizably human. But even this is just the start. It's just the movement of the painting. It no longer exists. Not in this form anyway. It's already imperceptible to the eye. There is no record, no visual tracking, no photographic memory. A history only those present will know. It's already on the journey to becoming something else. A self-portrait that recognizes its own disappearance. A complex background to the life that is already in existence and appearing before us in all its abstract colourations.

She takes a break and then returns. The art needs to breathe. It needs its time to reflect in its own de/re/composing. How do the colours feel when the artist is no longer present? Is there a secret life to paintings too? It already looks different from her. More mature, fuller of imperfections. They need to stay. It's the perfect lines that cause the most consternation. Even the clips that attach the canvas to the easel are haphazardly placed. Yellows and browns are now added, skinned hued tones for a layering of lightness that also resides in the heart of being. Seen from a different angle the work could now easily be read as a cloud formation of the mind. Or is it in the inner workings of a vital organ within? More yellow. Blacker. The mixing of the colours itself is an artform; yellows, browns, reds, purples, blacks, each with its own distinct character, merge together to deepen the sensibility from the edges. The most interesting characters always appear at the margins. The paint that is added always comes from the outside, and its results are never certain. It's an experiment. Never exact, yet that too is part of the artistic process. The colour is felt into existence. So many possibilities vanish before the final one is settled upon. Until the next layer that is. A change in light is necessary. How the slightest change in lighting makes a world of difference. The painter knows this, which is why they always distrust those who seek to manufacture neon wonderment or at least conceal the importance of glittering lights for a screened existence. As the detail is added, the lines appear finer. The line is more considered in its touch. Slower still. The rotations remain, but are less apparent, the shape of the emergent face more final perhaps in its lasting impressions. Contradictions abound. The lightness of touch adds tremendous weight, the slowness of movement adds intensity to the overall narrative from which the background is elevated. The shadow thus becomes us, not to cast a long burden over history, but to relieve us from the saving. Slower stiller. Just one more colour. Blue for now. A utopic promise? More the wilderness of the mind! Then the white. A centred touch of hope? A spiritual marking for a poetic time to come? Or a sinister digital signature and a reminder of the new tormentors in our midst?

The language of connection is futile here. You don't connect with these artistic lines or their movements of feeling. They take you on an unknown journey instead. Yes, they are welcoming. Yes, they are immersive. And yes, they may ask deeper questions about the pretence of being in the company of something that belongs to the Other. But these lines are literally good for nothing. A nothing that means something if something is meant to be. Still, what is the use of such lines then if they don't connect us? A technocrat may counter here and explain there is no art on an extinct planet. The lines shadowing this portrait tell a different story. Without the machines, there would be no extinction. Again, this is not a testimony. Though it does testify to the exceptionalism of being human. They testify without confession. Contours of a life that is tired of just trying to escape. Besides, what is the use of a line of flight anyway when there is nowhere left to fly to? It is patently wrong to see abstract art as a means of escaping from 'the world'. What is this world we speak of? Such a claim relegates again the abstract to the realm of the unreal. The abstract is as much of this world as the deep red apple that refuses to fall downward from the majestic tree that is also aware of its own ancestral singularity. Lines reveal to us the traces of an existence, which still exist on their own terms. That is also why the critical focus in art on 'vanishing points' somewhat misses the point. The vanishing is there the moment the lines appear. It originates from a void that is the only theory of ontology worthy of our lasting consideration. A void we may add that through the appearance of the line makes us realize nobody is in control. What matters instead is the ecology of the self, which appreciates the singularity of the line and its place in history. If everything flees, then nothing remains. If nothing remains, then only the void is present. The latter we can agree upon. But not every abstract line is intent upon its escape. Some instead would have us deliberate more on the depths of the void that are present everywhere, especially within. Lines in other words which are barely moving, yet full of distinct promise for the intricacies of experience they paint for us. Lines so intense they evoke a beautiful silence so that conversation is ripped

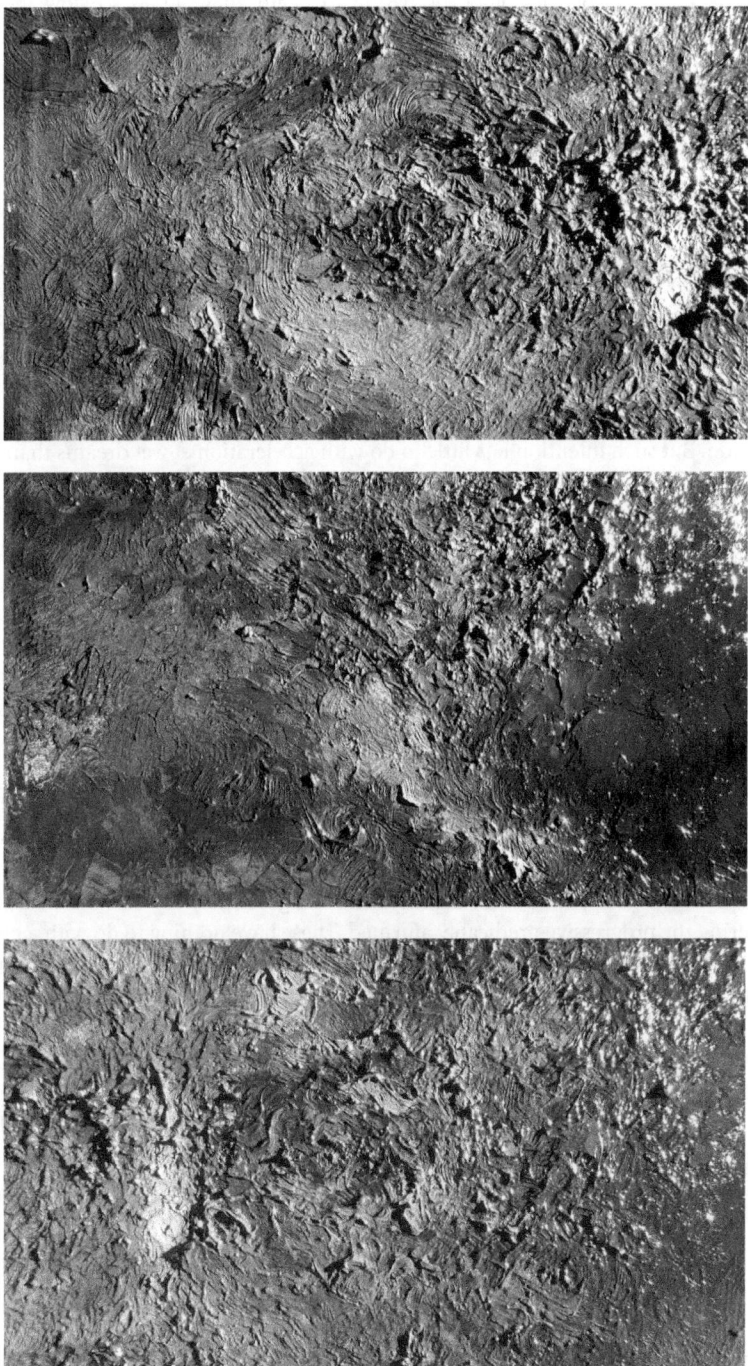

Figures 2.2, 2.3 and 2.4 Artwork: Chantal Meza, *Details from Self Portrait*, 2021. Oil on canvas, 55 × 66 cm. © Chantal Meza.

from the sacred throne to allow discussion to begin anew. Lines so slow in their movements it's easy to miss how their subtle gestures can appear as marginally central as they are free.

This brings us to the question of resistance, which requires us to further address the issues of intensity and the line of flight. Deleuze and Guattari begin their chapter in *A Thousand Plateaus* on imperceptibility with their concern with the intensity of becoming. Such intensification is bound to their idea of the haecceity, which can be explained as 'pure relations of speeds and slowness, nothing else'.[27] Though as we would expect, these are not so determined as they also envisage a 'slowness' that is able to be 'transformed into the breakneck speed of our waiting'. Yet, as we see it, intensity has nothing whatsoever to do with speed or the ability to accelerate and slow the flows of life. It is in fact less about movement and more about atmosphere. Moreover, as the etymology would suggest, *int*ensity shares a notable affinity with *int*ention, which is realized in the act of its appearance. Like the technical, the poetic too reveals its own intention. But such intention has little to do with accelerationist wet dreams than with the fires of a deeper contemplation, which intensifies atmospheric states of being while things are slowed down. This is not about inaction. On the contrary, it's all about creating the conditions of the new. A vision of what truly matters, which only gives secondary importance to the speed of flows. Just think of the most intense moments in sport; they occur in the moment just before the ball is hit. Or the most intense moments in music; they are found in the pauses that allow us to contemplate the heights and depths. And what of the most intense moments in life? Are they not belonging to the nocturnal silences of pre-immanent affective states that puncture the air in anticipation of what is to come? Such an understanding allows us to appreciate the importance of the *intensive contemplative act* that moves to an entirely different rhythm. It belongs to a different composition from the now familiar hyper-aroused performances of digital immersion, which is full of background noise, accelerates everything and yet creates nothing anew. Hyperactivity, hyperarousal and hyper-attentiveness are mere identarian positions for a world that has already been imagined and its technical lines for mastering the progressive predicably affirmed. These have nothing to do with a people to come than to bed down even further into the politics of survival and its inevitable theological clouding. Echoing Byung-Chul Han:

> We owe the cultural achievements of humanity – which include philosophy – to deep, contemplative attention. Culture presumes an environment in which deep attention is possible. Increasingly such immersion is being displaced by an entirely different form of attention: hyperattention. A rash of change of focus between different tasks, sources of information, and processes characterises this scattered mode of awareness. Since it also has a low tolerance for boredom, it does not admit the profound idleness that benefits the creative process. . . . A purely hectic rush produces nothing new.[28]

So, what of the new? It is now almost trite to say that, for Deleuzians' resistance is all about 'lines of flight'. While we find the idea of flight compelling (especially as it relates to air as imagined by Gaston Bachelard), not enough qualitative attention is given to the line. This brings us back to a distinction we have drawn between the poetic and the technical abstract as it relates directly to the line. Again, we agree with Deleuze and Guattari on the importance of the line. We also agree with them on the primacy of the abstract in terms of its creative expressiveness, while further subscribing to the notion that the abstract in thought is the thought of resistance. However, we don't see the line as being primarily concerned with flight. Maybe this is a problem of translation too. *Fuite* is not just about escape. It invokes a disappearance. It is all about the vanishing point, which make imperceptibility possible. So, yes, the abstract is the primary form of expression, and yes, the intention of the line matters. But the line, as we see it, cannot be so reduced, especially to a question of fleeing or escaping alone. The line reveals something deeper. The lines which Deleuze and Guattari paint are still too much bound to a surface, tied to the plane. Or when it comes to art, to paraphrase their critique of Chomksy, we suggest their thinking is 'both too abstract and not abstract enough'![29] Openly attuned to the machinic, they have inspiringly cut across terrains and had us purposefully focus upon the potentiality of unknown destinations. True, they imagine the 'above' and 'below', yet this is too easily absolved today. Instead, what if the line was already there, simply waiting to be revealed like the wound that existed before us? What if the line simply opens us a passage into the depths of the void, not an untimely gesture cutting across space, but cutting within the depths of time itself, to reveal the future to come? Certainly, understood this way, the intention of the cut would mean everything. It would also force us to confront the idea that with the abstract, it's not the line, which is of primary importance, but the intention to electrify the void.

Seeing the battle as one between poetic and technical imaginations allows us to provide more clarity on the relationship between technology and the state in the contemporary order of things. The state controls mass. Its focus remains bodies in space and time. The state policies the movement of bodies, segregates them into meaningful enclaves, while providing the illusion of politics so there is still a visible form to blame when things inevitably go wrong. This is its primary purpose, all the while reminding us that the world is ultimately insecure by design. Technology is all about the rule. It concerns the mapping, the monitoring and the controlling of each and every movement that exists within the confines of the state. But it is so much more than this. Unlike the poetic intuition that welcomes the unknown journey, flowing with the currents without the demand to determine, technology anticipates in advance and steers our behaviours through its affirmations and cancellations. Technology provides the culture. It shapes performance in unrivalled ways. It dictates the political, authenticating the rule of truth and the truth of rule. Technology arms the moralist with an unrequited progressivism. Sometimes this is done in the name of health and the saving of lives. Other times in making the world more aware of its wider ills. Both of which feed upon and further impress the absolute need for informational 'connectivity'. Technology as such is all about the creation of communities through a mastery of the line. It is the unrivalled creator of worlds that seeks to tame and invert the poetic cut. A persuasive colonizing machine that claims the void to be its own. It is then humanity's greatest theological achievement; indeed, it is (or so it is said) what ultimately makes humanity possible in the long run as it saves us from our own ruination. That is why technology is ultimately neuropolitical. It colonizes minds. It has become distinctly concerned with authoring the creative process, while suffocative of those intensively contemplative fires, which allows autonomous forms of creation to thrive in countenance to technological visions of species being. Without technology, we are told, there is no humanity, there is no progress, and there is no hope. Just as there is no art and therefore no future! Technology then is not just about immanence. It takes hold of projections in time. So, yes, the state still matters. But only as a means for controlling bodies and rendering them sedentary in ways that take us far beyond the striation of space critiqued by Deleuze and Guattari. And, yes, control still concerns, but it's far more pervasive than the authors ever imagined.

We know there is no escape. We are fully immersed. We are already living a transhumanist existence. Does that mean we are defeated? Perhaps. But we must still try, still fight to retain something of the human in this world. Yet if we might call upon the line today, it must be a line that reveals the poetic abstract anew. A line that is aware of its own abstract becoming in relation to the void, its own relation to the unknown, its own effacement. Such a line dances. Gil Anidjar reminds us here that to d-ance opens that precise in-between space in and through the grammar of one's own disappearance.[30] It is a line which proposes no hierarchy but is exceptional all the same. A line that moves to an ancestral beat, keeping hold of the secret as it imagines the fiery manes of horses, the likes conjured by the poet and songwriter Nick Cave. Cave laments a time when imagination is stripped bare by positivism, truth and science. Cave is arguably the most important poet for these times, often crafting words and sculpting sounds that echo deep and beyond in the infinity of the void. But Cave also pays his due respects. None more so than with his own Cosmic Dance that has nothing to do with some public spectacle, than to invoke a deeply intimate and solitary being after death that finds company in the beautiful and strident lyrics of Mark Bolan, who danced himself into the tomb, and asked how strange it was to consider whether he was dancing so soon? The pandemic has made a technological tomb of us all. It's time we learned to dance again with a contemplative intensity that dreams as it flies in the lightning storm of our own wilderness. A dance which has nothing to do with mimesis or imitation. A dance which has no desire to be in with the times and the comforts of a rehearsed orchestration. A dance instead that replaces connectivity with composition, replaces speed with contemplation: dancing alone because the dancer knows they are already in the company of ghosts.

Notes

1 See Gilles Deleuze and Felix Guattari, *A Thousand Plateaus* (London, Continuum: 2004).
2 This claim is first made in Brad Evans, *Ecce Humanitas: Beholding the Pain of Humanity* (New York, Columbia University Press: 2021). It is further elaborated in Brad Evans and Chantal Meza, 'The Techno-Theodicy: How Technology Became the New Religion' (*Theory & Event*, forthcoming).
3 Gilles Deleuze, 'Postscript on the Societies of Control' (October, Vol. 59: 1992) pp. 3–7.
4 This idea was properly articulated nearly three decades ago in Manuel Castells, *The Rise of the Networked Society: The Information Age: Economy, Society and Culture, Vol. I* (Oxford, Blackwell Publishers: 1996).

5 Michael Hardt and Antonio Negri, *Empire* (New England, Harvard University Press: 2000).
6 Zygmunt Bauman, *Society under Siege* (Cambridge, Polity Press: 2002).
7 Michael Dillon and Julian Reid, *The Liberal Way of War*; and Julian Reid, *The Biopolitics of the War on Terror: Life Struggles, Liberal Modernity and the Defense of Logistical Societies* (Manchester, Manchester University Press: 2006).
8 Jean Baudrillard, 'From the Universal to the Singular: The Violence of the Global', in Jérôme Bindé (ed.) *The Future of Values: 21st-Century Talks* (New York, UNESCO/ Bergen: 2004) p. 21.
9 Slavoj Žižek, *Organs without Bodies: Deleuze & Consequences* (London, Routledge, 2004).
10 Brad Evans, *Liberal Terror* (Cambridge, Polity Press: 2013).
11 This was duly noted by Giorgio Agamben at the height of the pandemic in a short mediation on facelessness. The prose is available online at: https://autonomies.org/2021/05/giorgio-agamben-on-the-government-of-the-faceless-and-the-deathless/
12 On this see Adriana Cavarero, *Horrorism: Naming Contemporary Violence* (New York, Columbia University Press: 2007).
13 Deleuze and Guattari, *Thousand Plateaus* p. 168.
14 Deleuze and Guattari, *Thousand Plateaus* p. 280.
15 This point is made explicitly in Evans, *Ecce Humanitas*.
16 While there is considerable research on this, see especially Wendy Chun, *Discriminating Data: Correlation, Neighbourhoods, and the New Politics of Recognition* (Boston, MIT Press: 2021).
17 See Brad Evans and Julian Reid, *Resilient Life: The Art of Living Dangerously* (Cambridge, Polity Press: 2014).
18 Paul Virilio, *The Vision Machine* (Bloomington and London, Indiana University Press and British Film Institute: 1994) p. 13.
19 Brad Evans and Chantal Meza, 'Violence & Abstraction' (*Symploke*, Vol. 29 No. 1: 2021) pp. 333–361.
20 Deleuze and Guattari, *Thousand Plateaus* pp. 286–287.
21 See especially on this Marshall McLuhan, *War & Peace in the Global Village* (Berkeley CA, Gingko Press: 1968).
22 Raymond Williams, *Modern Tragedy* (London, Vintage: 1966).
23 Raymond Williams, *Television: Technology and Cultural Form* (London, Fontana: 1974).
24 Williams, *Television: Technology and Cultural Form* p. 133.
25 Online at: https://lareviewofbooks.org/article/the-computer-says-what/
26 On this see, Brad Evans and Chantal Meza 'Immersive: A Violent Interruption to a Visual Silence' (*Washington University Review of Philosophy* Vol. 2: 2022).
27 Deleuze and Guattari, *Thousand Plateaus* p. 271.
28 Byung-Chul Han, *The Burnout Society* (Stanford, Stanford University Press: 2015) p. 13.
29 Deleuze and Guattari, *Thousand Plateaus* p. 148.
30 Gil Anidjar, 'D-ance' in Brad Evans and Chantal Meza (eds.) *State of Disappearance* (Montreal, McGill-Queens University Press: 2023).

References

Agamben, G. (2021, 4 May), *On the Government of the Faceless and the Deathless*. Autonomies. Retrieved 5 September 2022, from https://autonomies.org/2021/05/giorgio-agamben-on-the-government-of-the-faceless-and-the-deathless/

Anidjar, G. (2023), D-ance. In B. Evans and C. Meza (Eds.), *State of Disappearance*. Essay, Montreal: McGill-Queens University Press.

Baudrillard, J. (2004), From the Universal to the Singular: The Violence of the Global. In Bindé Jérôme (Ed.), *The Future of Values: 21st-Century Talks*. Essay, New York: UNESCO/Bergen.

Bauman, Z. (2002), *Society under Siege*. Cambridge: Polity Press.

Castells, M. (1996), *The Rise of the Networked Society* (Vol. 1, Ser. The Information Age: Economy, Society and Culture). Oxford: Blackwell Publishers.

Cavarero, A. (2007), *Horrorism: Naming Contemporary Violence*. (W. McCuaig, Trans.). New York: Columbia University Press.

Chun, W. (2021), *Discriminating Data: Correlation, Neighborhoods, and the New Politics of Recognition*. Boston: MIT Press.

Deleuze, G. (1992), Postscript on the Societies of Control. *October*, *59*, 3–7. http://www.jstor.org/stable/778828

Deleuze, G., and Guattari, F. (2004), *A Thousand Plateaus: Capitalism and Schizophrenia*. (B. Massumi, Trans.). London: Continuum.

Dicken, P. (2021, 13 September), The Computer Says . . . What? *Los Angeles Review of Books*. Retrieved 5 September 2022, from https://lareviewofbooks.org/article/the-computer-says-what/

Dillon, M., and Reid, J. (2009), *The Liberal Way of War: Killing to Make Life Live*. London: Routledge.

Evans, B. (2013), *Liberal Terror*. Cambridge: Polity Press.

Evans, B. (2021), *Ecce Humanitas: Beholding the Pain of Humanity*. New York: Columbia University Press.

Evans, B., and Meza, C. (2021), Violence and Abstraction. *Symploke*, *29*(1–2), 333–361. https://doi.org/10.1353/sym.2021.0018

Evans, B., and Meza, C. (2022), Immersive: A Violent Interruption to a Visual Silence. *Washington University Review of Philosophy*, *2*, 219–235. https://doi.org/10.5840/wurop2022214

Evans, B., and Meza, C. (2022), The Techno-Theodicy: How Technology Became the New Religion. *Theory & Event*, *25*(3), 639–664. https://doi.org/10.1353/tae.2022.0031

Evans, B., and Reid, J. (2014), *Resilient Life: The Art of Living Dangerously*. Cambridge: Polity Press.

Han, Byung-Chul. (2015), *The Burnout Society*. (E. Butler, Trans.). Stanford: Stanford University Press.

Hardt, M., and Negri, A. (2000), *Empire*. New England: Harvard University Press.

McLuhan, M., and Fiore, Q. (1968), *War and Peace in the Global Village*. Berkeley CA: Gingko Press.

Reid, J. (2006), *The Biopolitics of the War on Terror: Life Struggles, Liberal Modernity and the Defence of Logistical Societies*. Manchester: Manchester University Press.

Virilio, P. (1994), *The Vision Machine*. Bloomington and London: Indiana University Press and British Film Institute.

Williams, R. (1966), *Modern Tragedy*. London: Vintage.

Williams, R. (1974), *Television: Technology and Cultural Form*. London: Fontana.

Žižek Slavoj. (2004), *Organs without Bodies: Deleuze and Consequences*. London: Routledge.

3

Obscura Sacrificia: Covid and Neoliberalism

Brent Adkins

In Deleuze and Guattari's discussion of the war machine they describe it arriving suddenly between the two poles of sovereignty. Kleist illustrates this perfectly in his *Penthesilea* when the Amazon army arrives without warning in the middle of the Trojan and Greek armies arrayed for battle. While it is evident that Deleuze and Guattari invent the concept of the war machine to discuss its relation to the state, in this chapter I am interested in the collision between two war machines: a virus and neoliberal capitalism. In order to think through this collision I want to take up the story of Iphigeneia from the Epic Cycle. The details and ambiguities surrounding this story will illustrate two crucial points. First, the interaction between two war machines is the site of sacrifice. Second, the sacrifice is obscured. I will argue that the same logic of sacrifice and its obfuscation is operative in the response to the global pandemic under neoliberal capitalism.

Two war machines

The Achaeans are a war machine. They flow liquid over the Aegean to assail the walled city of Troy. Agamemnon holds the war bands together through the promise of glory and wealth. Homer's account of the war in the *Iliad* focuses heavily on the circulation of affect. It begins with Achilles' wrath, which interacts with Agamemnon's jealousy and Odysseus' cunning. Achilles broods while the tides of war turn against the Greeks. The Greeks, however, are not the only war machine at work in the Epic Cycle. The gods do not sit idly by. They, too, have their jealousies, pride and rivalries and often use human events as the site for their expression. Apollo sends a plague on the Greeks to force the return of Chryseis to her father. Artemis is offended by Agamemnon's claim that he is the greater hunter and stalls the entire fleet at Aulis.

Artemis exemplifies the smooth space created by the gods. A god of the trackless forest, she has no permanent home. She hunts. She remains unmarried and jealously guards her virginity. Acteon was turned into a stag and hunted by his own dogs for the crime of surprising Artemis while bathing. Now Agamemnon has roused Artemis' anger, not by threatening her virginity but by diminishing her skill with a bow. For this crime Agamemnon is not challenged to a test of skill (as with Arachne and Athena).

Rather, Artemis envelops the fleet in a stifling calm (or a contrary wind in some versions). The Greeks can neither move forward nor return home. They can no longer use the wind to smooth the space between them and the Trojans. While this encounter can easily be read as a conflict between two states (Greek and divine) or even as a conflict between a state and the war machine (divine and Greek), I think it is best read as an encounter between two war machines. The Greeks are not striated by their encounter with Artemis. They are not divided in order to be numbered. They are not treated as an extensive magnitude to be organized. They are becalmed. Artemis has turned the port of Aulis into a Sargasso Sea, a zero degree of intensity.

Calchas, mantis and priest, has divined not only that Artemis is the source of the Greek becalment but that the solution lies in the sacrifice of his daughter Iphigeneia. There is a complex analogy of proportion at work here by which the virgin Artemis had her sacred grove violated by the killing of one of her deer. The killer then had the temerity to boast that not even Artemis herself could have made such a shot. The analogy of proportion at work here, then, equates Artemis' virginity to the inviolability of her grove to the sacredness of her deer to the integrity of her reputation. In order to propitiate for this series of transgressions Calchas concludes that virgin blood must be spilled.[1] The sacrifice of Agamemnon's daughter is the natural completion of the series. Other sacrifices might seem more just to us. Why shouldn't Agamemnon himself bear the punishment of his transgressions? Or, why not abandon the war altogether and 'sacrifice' Helen? Or, why not offer Artemis another deer? None of these alternatives, however, completes the series. Thus, Agamemnon is left with an impossible choice:

> And then the elder monarch spake aloud-
> Ill lot were mine, to disobey!
> And ill, to smite my child, my household's love and pride!
>
> Aeschylus, *Agamemnon*, 249–251

It is important to note two things about Calchas' 'solution'. First, Artemis herself never clarifies her wishes in the matter. This is solely Calchas' determination. Second, regardless of Artemis' wishes, the sacrifice works. After the sacrifice the calm is lifted, and favourable winds take the Greeks to Troy.

The encounter between two war machines cannot be thought, though, as a simple summative or subtractive process. War machines are intensive, and intensities do not function like extensive magnitudes. Rather, Deleuze and Guattari suggest a process by which intensities envelope or are enveloped in other intensities. 'Exactly like a speed or a temperature, which is not composed of other speeds and temperatures but rather is *enveloped in or envelops* others, each of which marks a change in nature' (ATP 31, emphasis added). For example, if I have a 100 ml water at 20°C and I add 10 ml at 10°C, the resulting 110 ml of water is not 30°C. Intensities such as temperature are not additive in this way. Experience tells us that the overall temperature of the new volume will be slightly lower. In Deleuze and Guattari's terms, the larger volume of water envelops the added water. The result is water that is no longer 20°C or 10°C, but a new intensity altogether, albeit one mostly determined by the larger volume of water.

The Greeks at Aulis become enveloped by Artemis. This results in a complete change in their intensity. Aeschylus describes the Greek languishing in this way:

> And rife with ill delay
> From northern Strymon blew the thwarting blast-
> Mother of famine fell,
> That holds men wand'ring still
> Far from the haven where they fain would be!-
> And pitiless did waste
> Each ship and cable, rotting on the sea,
> And, doubling with delay each weary hour,
> Withered with hope deferred th' Achaeans' warlike flower.
>
> *Agamemnon*, 236–243

In Aulis everything becomes subject to a wasting away. The soldiers waste away from hunger. The ships begin to rot. Perhaps worst of all the 'warlike flower' of the Greeks begins to wither. Agamemnon and Menelaus understand that this change in intensity will be fatal for their plans to besiege Troy. Furthermore, they will never be able to muster such an army again. They consult Calchas on the matter, whose solution seems absurd if the problem is extensive, but plausible from the perspective of intensities. The sacrifice of Iphigeneia is an attempt to introduce enveloping intensities into the encounter between two war machines. Agamemnon's pride is humbled. Artemis' wrath is cooled. The Greeks shift from depressed to joyful. The calm becomes a westerly wind headed towards Troy. None of these shifts in intensity occurs, though, because joy or humility or even wind is 'added'. Rather, the sacrifice is a division that changes the relation of all the intensities to one another. It is an event that sets the intensities into a different relation from one another.

Even though the shift in intensities arises from the sacrifice, a profound ambiguity remains with regard to the sacrifice itself. Was Iphigeneia sacrificed, or not? Was she killed on the altar or replaced by a stag at the last minute? Both versions of the story are found throughout the Greek and Latin literary canons. Euripides saves Iphigeneia, while Aeschylus does not. Ovid repeats Euripides' version of events, while Lucretius follows Aeschylus. The narrative advantage to Iphigeneia actually being sacrificed is that it sets in motion the cycle of revenge and death when Clytemnestra kills Agamemnon and then Orestes kills Clytemnestra. The theological advantage of replacing Iphigeneia with a stag at the last second is that it avoids imputing the horror of human sacrifice to Artemis. Or, at least it shows Artemis' mercy at the last minute and her protection of the innocent.

In sum, then, the confrontation between two war machines cannot be thought as aggregation. Rather, Deleuze and Guattari suggest that such an encounter results in logic of envelopment. This logic differs from the aggregative logic of extensities and suggests that meeting of intensities results in a change in both intensities. At the site of the encounter we find a sacrifice that's both necessary and unacknowledged. The victim is divine for being both an object of sacrifice and being spared from sacrifice. In Euripides' telling Iphigeneia is whisked away to Tauris to become a priestess of Artemis.

Her absence whether by death or divine intervention confers divinity. It is her reward for occupying the liminal space between two war machines. The logic of envelopment is the logic of sacrifice, but precisely because envelopment changes the nature of the intensities involved, the sacrifice is forgotten.

Neoliberalism as a war machine

Deleuze and Guattari do not identify capitalism as a war machine until *A Thousand Plateaus*. However, beginning in *Anti-Oedipus* they argue that the operations of capitalism are distinct from the operations of the state or society. While both society and the state operate according to codes and territories, capitalism operates according to an axiomatic. A great deal, then, hinges on this distinction between codes and axioms. For Deleuze and Guattari a code has three primary characteristics: 'indirect, qualitative, and limited' (AO 247). In contrast to this axioms are direct, quantitative and unlimited, as well as having the fourth characteristic of privatizing the public as a consequence of the first three (AO 251).

In order to clarify what is at stake in the shift from codes to axioms and its connection to a war machine, let's take a look at these characteristics individually. Why are codes indirect while axioms are direct? Codes are Deleuze and Guattari's way of talking about reality as a semiotic process. Desiring production produces its own limit (the body without organs), which causes desiring production to fall back on itself and spread out across the body without organs. This process of falling back and spreading across is called recording. The recording process captures desiring production as signs or as coded (AO 38–40). It's important to note at this point that neither signs nor codes is to be taken in a linguistic sense. Language is a code, but not all codes are linguistic. Codes are not even fundamentally human. The relation between a wasp and an orchid that attracts it is coded. Even the way that sediments deposited by a river are sorted by size and density is a code for Deleuze and Guattari. *Anti-Oedipus* thus presents us with a metaphysics of flows and a process for their coding. These coded flows are heterogeneous and interact with other flows in complex and non-linear ways. The coding of flows is also precisely what makes their interaction indirect rather than direct.

To illustrate how this indirection works let's return to Deleuze and Guattari's discussion of the non-state and state social formations. Borrowing language from Levi-Strauss, they argue that coding in these societies is captured in two irreducible flows, filiation and alliance.[2] Filiation concerns the coding of lines of descent and concerns questions of kinship relation. What degree of cousins may marry, for example? Alliance concerns the coding of other social relations. Who may hunt? At what age? What rituals are required? Even though both codings apply to everyone in society they are not equal or interchangeable. Their relation must always be negotiated. In a non-state society these negotiations are complex and may require adjudication from several sources. In a state society all of the codes are overcoded so that they pass through the king or central authority. The codes may forbid and allow exactly the same interactions as before, but now all is done under the aegis of the king who is seen as the origin and end of all codes in the state. Notice, however, that even in the state code remains indirect, but the indirection is mediated through the king.

Deleuze and Guattari give little indication of the origin of the term 'axiom' in their work. The reference to the work of the Bourbaki group suggests a mathematical (though not Euclidean) use of the term. 'Bourbaki says as much concerning scientific axiomatics: they do not form a Taylor system, nor a mechanical game of isolated formulas, but rather imply "intuitions" that are linked to resonances and conjunctions of structures, and that are merely aided by the "powerful levers" of technique' (AO 251). Guattari further confirms this in the *Anti-Oedipus Papers*: 'The idea of a scientific task that no longer passes through codes but rather through an axiomatic first took place in mathematics toward the end of the nineteenth century.... One finds this well formed only in the capitalism of the nineteenth century' (22 February, 1972). 'Axiom' in the sense deployed here appears to be ad hoc and experimental, a way of grouping or conjoining flows that supports the original intuitions. This means that axioms are neither a priori nor finite. Rather, they are continually invented. This is in stark contrast to codes that are always bound up in semiotic chains. Of course codes change and develop, but they cannot be freely invented.

As we saw above, codes interact indirectly. In contrast to this axioms work directly on decoded flows. The first implication of this is that while the functioning of codes depends on their irreducibility and non-equivalence, axioms make everything exchangeable with everything else. Capitalist axiomatics does this by making everything exchangeable for money.

> By substituting money for the very notion of a code, it has created an axiomatic of abstract quantities that keeps moving further and further in the direction of the deterritorialization of the socius. Capitalism tends toward a threshold of decoding that will destroy the socius in order to make it a body without organs and unleash the flows of desire on this body as a deterritorialized field (AO 33).

In essence capitalism takes all of the non-economic relations that are traditionally governed by irreducible codes of alliance and filiation and decodes them by introducing money as a universal solution in which all codes are dissolved.

By precisely the same means the qualitative distinction between alliance and filiation is replaced with a quantitative distinction measured in terms of economic value. Differences in kind are replaced by differences in degree under a capitalist axiomatic. Finally, while indirect relations and qualitative distinctions limit the possibilities for interactions among codes, axiomatics are unlimited. Not only is everything in principle exchangeable, but an axiomatic system actively seeks to expand its horizons. Finding new markets, filling new needs, the bedrock of entrepreneurial capitalism continually invents new axioms in order to expand the reach of capitalism.

Though Deleuze and Guattari do not use the term 'neoliberalism', it is clear that they have identified its salient features. In *A Thousand Plateaus* they identify capitalism with a war machine precisely because it functions by decoding and deterritorialization. They further identify there the ways that global economy forces states to function at the behest of capitalism rather than the other way around. The contemporary situation, then, is one in which capitalism deploys the state rather than the state capturing the war machine. 'In principle, all States are isomorphic; in other words, they are domains of realization of capital as a function of a sole external world market' (ATP 464). Different state forms may differ in the way that they code the socius. They may even differ in whether they multiply capitalist axioms (as in social democracies) or subtract axioms (as in more restrictive forms of government), but all states must participate in the same global market. States are no longer distinct from the market, they are 'domains of realization of capital'. It is this absorption of the state into the market that is the hallmark of neoliberalism and explains the global response to the pandemic.

Covid as a war machine

Viruses form an important touchstone throughout *A Thousand Plateaus*. For Deleuze and Guattari viruses are emblematic of the kind of becomings that they are trying to think. Whereas traditionally philosophy has characterized becomings that proceed from one essential being to another in a linear, filiative fashion, viruses show the material reality of non-linear, non-filiative becomings that traverse beings and compose rhizomes through heterogeneous connections. A virus, for example, can connect a baboon and a cat at the cellular level (ATP 10). Becoming is thus not subordinated to being on a genealogical model of reproduction. Rather, becoming itself is thought as creative.

Deleuze and Guattari expand their analysis of becoming as viral in two ways. In the first instance, they say that viral becomings are essential to all becomings-animal. This fits well with their insistence the becoming-animal is in no way related to imitation. Imitation subordinates becoming to being and merely seeks reproduction. In contrast to this becoming-animal is affective and intensive and seeks the circulation of some affects and the exclusion of others. Slepian does not put shoes on his hands in order to imitate a dog. He puts shoes on his hands so that the intensities of having opposable thumbs will be excluded and he will have to comport himself differently in the world (ATP 258–259). It is precisely because becoming involves intensities that contagion, rather than reproduction, is the better way of conceiving it. Deleuze and Guattari write:

> The difference is that contagion, epidemic, involves terms that are entirely heterogeneous: for example, a human being, an animal, and a bacterium, a virus, a molecule, a microorganism. Or in the case of the truffle, a tree, a fly, and a pig. These combinations are neither genetic nor structural; they are interkingdoms, unnatural participations. That is the only way Nature operates – against itself. This is a far cry from filiative production or hereditary reproduction (ATP 242).

Viral becomings thus provide a way for Deleuze and Guattari to think about nature as composed of heterogeneous rhizomes as opposed to discrete, molar entities. Through the human–Covid rhizome the entire world has embarked on a becoming that, while its long-term effects are as yet unknown, its immediate short-term effects were a massive reduction in economic intensity. Economies shrank. Traffic eased. Pollution abated. People died.

The second way that Deleuze and Guattari deploy the viral is in a political register. In 'Micropolitics and Segmentarity', the primary task is to give an account of fascism. Their analysis shows that fascism must not be thought as a species of totalitarianism, but rather as an intensive and affective micropolitics that operates on the molecular level and may or may not coalesce on the molar level. Deleuze and Guattari write:

> As we have seen, microfascisms have a specificity of their own that can crystallize into a macrofascism, but may also float along the supple line on their own account and suffuse every little cell. A multitude of black holes may very well not become centralized, and acts instead as viruses adapting to the most varied situations, sinking voids in molecular perceptions and semiotics. Interactions without resonance (ATP 228).

Here microfascism is pictured as a contagion that produces voids or black holes around which intensities circulate. What Deleuze and Guattari have in mind here are the unassailable beliefs and presuppositions that form the foundations of our judgements. They continue:

> Instead of the great paranoid fear, we are trapped in a thousand little monomanias, self-evident truths, and clarities that gush from every black hole and no longer form a system, but are only rumble and buzz, blinding lights giving any and everybody the mission of self-appointed judge, dispenser of justice, policeman, neighborhood SS man. We have overcome fear, we have sailed from the shores of security, only to enter a system that is no less concentricized, no less organized: the system of petty insecurities that leads everyone to their own black hole in which to turn dangerous, possessing a clarity on their situation, role, and mission even more disturbing than the certitudes of the first [rigidly segmented] line (ATP 228).

From this vantage point we can glimpse the source of the anger with which many have reacted to public health measures during the pandemic. It's not that the anger has a single source; it's that these public health measures strike at the 'thousand little monomanias' that have been installed as our center of gravity. Public health attempts to segment these black holes and the response has been to maintain them at any cost. In the United States these monomanias have begun to resonate together under the banner of QAnon, which connects a wildly disparate set of economic, political, racial, social and cultural concerns under the banner of fighting an unseen but implacable enemy. This is how microfascism becomes macrofascism.

> But fascism is inseparable from a proliferation of molecular focuses in interaction, which skip from point to point, before beginning to resonate together in the National Socialist State. Rural fascism and city or neighborhood fascism, youth fascism and war veteran's fascism, fascism of the Left and fascism of the Right, fascism of the couple, family, school, and office: every fascism is defined by a

> micro-black hole that stands on its own and communicates with the others, before resonating in a great, generalized central black hole. There is fascism when a war machine is installed in each hole, in every niche (ATP 214).

Those in support of public health mandates are often baffled by the ferocity leveled against their enforcement. Suddenly, the problem of quarantining, masking and vaccines is related to gun rights, freedom, politics, voting laws and the Black Lives Matter protests. Critical Race Theory is now the current object of ire among those opposed to public health mandates. When the furor over Critical Race Theory dies down it will be replaced by something new. In every case, while the putative object of outrage is new, its true source will always be traced to the shadowy enemy within. What many arguing against this manufactured outrage miss is that its origins are molecular. While the debate happens at the molar level of policy, the policy is incidental to the intensive affects circulating at the molecular level.

From this perspective we can organize the various responses to the pandemic in terms of Covid as a war machine seeking to decode and deterritorialize the state and enveloping intensities at various levels from biological populations to the global economy. The response of the state to a war machine is always to capture it. The state sought to capture it in numerous ways from overcoding to striation. The process of overcoding involved naming the disease, tracing its origin, and ultimately producing a vaccine. Striation included public health policies such as testing, quarantining, masking, restricting travel and social distancing. This multi-pronged attack was an attempt to capture and neutralize something that could not be stopped, precisely because viral transmission is transversal and heterogeneous rather than linear and homogeneous. Covid's airborne transmission vector smoothed the striated space of the state.

Envelopment: Covid and neoliberalism

While much work remains to be done in relation to the state and microfascist responses to Covid, my primary concern here is the response of neoliberal capitalism. Here I would like to return to the parallels that can be drawn with the story of Iphigeneia. As we saw above, the story can be read not simply as the conflict between two states, the Greeks and the gods, each seeking to striate the other, but rather as the conflict between two war machines, the marauding pack of sailors and the goddess of the hunt, the sea and the forest. At Aulis Artemis envelops the sea and threatens to transform it into a placid, woodland lake. In the same way the spread of Covid enveloped the global economy and radically reduced its intensity. The reduction in intensity, however, was not uniform. Unlike the Iphigeneia story, though, Covid does not directly cause the reduction in economic intensity; it is the state through travel restrictions and quarantines. Here I think a more complex story could be told about the relation between the organic and the linguistic strata. In this case Covid and neoliberalism are deterritorializing edges of their respective strata, each attempting to envelop the other. State reactions to Covid are attempts by the linguistic stratum to overcode the organic and reach their pinnacle in the development of a vaccine. In the Iphigeneia story state intervention is religious intervention. The state's solution to envelopment by a war machine is striation. Here religious ritual striates the smooth space. As we saw above, Calchas works through the complex series of proportion and arrives at the conclusion that propitiation can only occur through the sacrifice of Iphigeneia. Her blood will inoculate the Greeks against the wrath of Artemis and the transgression of Agamemnon's hubris.

Iphigeneia's sacrifice and its obfuscation brings us to the point of closest proximity with the Covid pandemic. Not only is the literary tradition surrounding Iphigeneia divided against itself, it also portrays Iphigeneia in two distinct ways. In the tradition codified by Aeschylus Iphigeneia is a mute victim tricked into her sacrifice, surprised and terrified by her fate. This portrayal runs up against the longstanding tradition in the ancient world that sacrificial animals must go willingly to their deaths.[3] In contrast to this, Euripides makes Iphigeneia a more pious sacrifice by having her willingly accept her sacrifice.

> But the maid, standing close by her father, spoke thus: 'O my father, here I am; willingly I offer my body for my country and all Hellas, that you may lead me to the altar of the goddess and sacrifice me, since this is Heaven's ordinance. May good luck be yours for any help that I afford! and may you obtain the victor's gift and come again to the land of your fathers. So then let none of the Argives lay hands on me, for I will bravely yield my neck without a word' (*Iphigenia at Aulis*, 1550–1559).

During the initial stages of the pandemic both versions of Iphigeneia's sacrifice played out simultaneously. Many willingly risked exposure to the virus in order to maintain what the US Department of Homeland Security called 'critical infrastructure'. Concomitant to defining critical infrastructure as the maintenance of the public health, security and economy of the country was the creation of the category of 'essential worker'. In some respects there is a homology between the divinity of the sacrificial victim and the essentiality of the essential worker. Both are defined by the state. Both are identified according to the same analogy of proportion. Finally, both occupy the liminal space between two war machines. In the case of the pandemic, war metaphors abounded. Essential workers were 'on the front lines' or 'in the trenches'.

Though in some accounts of the Iphigeneia story Clytemnestra points out that Agamemnon can simply abandon Helen and there would be no need to fight the war, this never seems to be seriously considered. Agamemnon considers himself duty bound to the gods and Menelaus to prosecute this war. In the same way, a complete global shutdown for two weeks could have stopped the pandemic, but it was never seriously considered. Instead the loudest and most immediate cries came from those worried about the economy. 'The cure can't be worse than the disease' was a common talking point. Many reasoned that if we stopped the economy the consequences would be so dire that life would not be worth living in such a world. It's as if we were globally asked the robber's question, Your money or your life? and the majority chose money.

Some proposed that choosing money was in fact heroic. In the early months of the pandemic the Lt. Gov. of Texas, Dan Patrick, made the following remark: 'No one reached out to me and said, "as a senior citizen, are you willing to take a chance on your survival in exchange for keeping the America that all America loves for your children and grandchildren?"' Patrick continued, 'And if that's the exchange, I'm all in.' First of all, note that the sacrifice is articulated in purely economic terms, an exchange. It's as if his reasoning goes something like this: Given that people *must* die in order to save the economy, which people are the best candidates? By the same proportional logic that Calchas employed, Patrick reasons that it's old people who are the obvious candidates. They're the obvious candidates because they are the ones most at risk. Precisely because older people are at risk for Covid they should fully embrace this risk and work to ensure the smooth running of the economy. Second, note the metonymy operating between the state and the economy. While the context makes clear that Patrick is concerned with ending lockdown restrictions and 're-opening the country for business', he phrases this in terms of 'keeping the America that all America loves'. That is, maintaining America as a domain 'of realization of capital as a function of a sole external world market' (TP 464).

The willingness to sacrifice those most at risk became a clear but unacknowledged theme as the pandemic began to spread. Furthermore, since under neoliberalism states are not independent of the global economic market but functions of it, sacrifice is outsourced to exploited countries while vaccines are hoarded by exploiting countries. It is precisely on this point that Adorno and Horkheimer mistakenly locate the mechanics of capitalism in the tale of Odysseus and the sirens. While Odysseus listens to the irresistible beauty of the song without any risk, his men toil away heedlessly with their ears plugged with wax. Odysseus reaps the profit, which is extracted from the labour of his men. Indeed, if his men were to listen to the Siren song (that is, enjoy the profits of their labour), then all would be lost. Thus, on Adorno and Horkheimer's reading the myth of the Sirens shows not only the exploitative nature of capitalism but also the dire consequences of not allowing oneself to be exploited. There is exploitation here but no sacrifice.[4]

As we've seen, neoliberal capitalism requires continuous, ritualized sacrifice, while at the same time obscuring that sacrifice. We can see both the sacrifice and its occlusion in the two versions of the myth that arise in the Epic Cycle. In one version Iphigeneia is brutally slaughtered in order to ensure following winds for the Greek fleet travelling to Troy. In the other version Iphigeneia is spared at the last second when Artemis whisks her away and puts a golden stag in her place. In both cases the siege of Troy required the ritual of sacrifice, but in one telling the Greeks were unwilling to countenance the necessity of human sacrifice.

As Marx shows, human sacrifice is one of the hallmarks of capitalism. His descriptions of workers under capitalism are replete with references to hollowed out, undead creatures who do not fully possess themselves. This zombification has intensified under neoliberal capitalism as the global north extracts resources and labour from the global south. For the most part those living in the global north could live without acknowledging the sacrifices that their lives were predicated on. However, when the pandemic reached America there were immediate calls for people to voluntarily sacrifice themselves for the sake of the economy. The actual sacrifices, though, fell disproportionately on the service sectors, while at the same time these sacrifices were being disavowed by a large percentage of the population.

While the sacrifice of Iphigeneia may illustrate the logic at work here, it is Deleuze and Guattari's *Capitalism and Schizophrenia* that lays bare its mechanisms. Neoliberal capitalism is a war machine that exposes its suicidal tendencies when confronted by the war machine of a global pandemic as each tries to envelop the other.

Notes

1 See Deleuze and Guattari's discussion of analogies of proportion in *A Thousand Plateaus*, 234–237.
2 Levi-Strauss, *The Elementary Structures of Kinship*. Note that the French *filiation* is translated as 'descent' in Levi-Strauss but 'filiation' in *Anti-Oedipus*.
3 Walter Burkert, *Homo Necans: The Anthropology of Ancient Greek Sacrificial Ritual and Myth*, tr. by Peter Bing (Berkeley: University of California Press, 1986).
4 Adorno and Horkheimer, *The Dialectic of Enlightenment: Philosophical Fragments*, tr. by Edmund Jephcott (Stanford: Stanford University Press, 2002), 35–62.

References

Adorno, Theodor and Horkheimer, Max. *The Dialectic of Enlightenment: Philosophical Fragments*. tr. by Edmund Jephcott. Stanford: Stanford University Press, 2002.
Aeschylus. *Agamemnon* in *The Oresteia*. tr. by Robert Fagles. London: Penguin Books, 1984.
Burkert, Walter. *Homo Necans: The Anthropology of Ancient Greek Sacrificial Ritual and Myth*. tr. by Peter Bing. Berkeley: University of California Press, 1986.
Deleuze, Gilles and Guattari, Félix. *Anti-Oedipus: Capitalism and Schizophrenia, vol. 1*. tr. by Robert Hurley. Minneapolis: University of Minnesota Press, 1983.
Deleuze, Gilles and Guattari, Félix. *A Thousand Plateaus: Capitalism and Schizophrenia, vol. 2*. tr. by Brian Massumi. Minneapolis: University of Minnesota Press, 1987.
Euripides. *Iphigenia at Aulis* in *The Bacchae and Other Plays*. tr. by John Davie. London: Penguin Books, 2005.
Guattari, Félix. *The Anti-Oedipus Papers*. tr. by Kélina Gotman. New York: Semiotext(e), 2006.
Lévi-Strauss, Claude. *The Elementary Structures of Kinship*. tr. by James Harle Bell, et al. Boston: Beacon Press, 1969.

4

The Task of Thinking in The Age of Biopolitics: Between Heidegger and Deleuze

Tony See Sin Heng

Introduction

In 'The Invention of an Epidemic' (2020), the Italian philosopher Giorgio Agamben warned of the imminent rise of biopolitics during the COVID-19 global pandemic (Agamben 2020). The term 'biopolitics' refers to a political system that no longer sees human beings as having 'political life' but as 'bare life'. Therein the sole purpose of biopolitics is the expansion of power through the management of 'population'. He asks a simple question with regards to the manner in which the current global pandemic is managed: Why has the state been exaggerating the effects of the virus when it is clear that the high infection rate is accompanied by a disproportionately small death rate when compared with other infectious disease? To be sure, this does not mean that the virus is not fatal, it is just that the fatality is not necessary but *contingent* on some other pre-existing medical preconditions. Apparently, most of those who succumbed to the virus did so due to some prior conditions such as heart and kidney issues. If this is so, as Agamben pointed out, then 'why do the media and the authorities do their utmost to spread a state of panic, thus provoking in the authentic state of exception with serious limitations on movement and a suspension of daily life in entire regions?' Agamben suggests that this may be for the purpose of expanding the paradigm of biopolitics, or a state of exception, to all regions across the globe (Agamben 2020, 1).

The term 'biopolitics' is elaborated at length in Agamben's *Homo Sacer* (1998), where a distinction is made in juridico-political texts between 'political life' (*bios*) and 'bare life' (*zoe*). This relocates the human person from the justice system and firmly locates them within a zone of radical indistinction, where they can now be killed without violating either human or divine law (Agamben 1998, 81). In *State of Exception* (2005), it is found that this 'state of exception' did not wane with the rise of democratic political traditions but continued to expand when the idea of 'state of siege' was normalized, when police and military powers were authorized *at all times* in order to deal with 'internal sedition'. This logic of exception continued to expand across the globe when the president of the United States issued a 'military order' on 12 November 2001 which authorized the 'indefinite detention' of noncitizens who are suspected of involvement in terrorist activities. One consequence of this is that it effectively expanded the power of the attorney general, who was already invested with the power to 'take into custody' any alien suspected of activities that endangered 'the national security of the United States' by the USA Patriot Act issued on 26 October 2001.The irony of this is that citizens are now stripped of their rights in order to defend them from 'enemies' (Agamben 2005, 5).

One consequence of this is that 'the camp' becomes the new 'juridico-political paradigm' of the modern world (Agamben 1998, 169). Agamben states that 'The camp is the space of this absolute impossibility of deciding between fact and law, rule and application, exception and rule, which nevertheless incessantly decides between them' (1998, 173). When this camp is securely lodged within the city's interior, the camp can be seen as the new norm (*nomos*) of the modern (Agamben 1998, 174–175; 2000, 45). Thus, Agamben holds that asking how such atrocities could be committed against human beings misses the point and is 'hypocritical'; the real question to ask is how human beings could be so deprived of their rights that no act committed against them could be seen as a crime (Agamben 1998, 171; 2000, 41). If the essence of the camp consists in the appearance of a state of exception in space in which life and bare life enter into a threshold of indistinction, then the implication for this is that we must admit that we find ourselves in a camp every time such a structure is created (Agamben 1998, 174).

Agamben's recent book *Where Are We Now? The Epidemic As Politics* (2021) follows the overall trajectory of his thoughts on biopolitics. Agamben notes that one of the things that the global pandemic has brought about is the introduction of 'health' as a new 'religion' and a new function in national security. This means that health is increasingly weaponized, it has become a concept that is used to justify the power of the state, in what we may now call 'biosecurity'. It is interesting and important to remember how, at the beginning of the global pandemic, way before any vaccine was invented, the instruments of surveillance and social control were already almost everywhere in sight. This would suggest that the state is more obsessed with social control than with social safety from the virus. He says that this pandemic 'did not arrive unexpectedly' and that throughout history 'there are people and organizations pursuing licit or illicit objectives and then trying to realize those objectives by any means necessary' and '[f]or this reason, speaking of a conspiracy adds nothing to the reality of facts. Defining anyone who seeks to know historical events for what they really are as a "conspiracy theorist", however, is plain defamation' (Agamben, 2021, 75–76). The book concludes with the observation that we are moving towards the end of the old world, and the possible beginning of a new one. Agamben states:

> What is happening today on a global scale is certainly the end of a world. But it is not – as it is for those who are trying to govern in accordance with their own interests – an end in the sense of being a transition to a world that is better suited to the new needs of the human consortium. The era of bourgeois democracy, with its rights, its constitutions, and its parliaments, is fading. But beyond this surface level legal transformation, which is certainly not irrelevant, what is ending is, primarily, the world that began with the Industrial Revolution and built up to the two – or

> three – world wars and to the totalitarianisms – tyrannical or democratic – that accompanied them (Agamben 2021, 96).

The idea of 'biopolitics' is, to be sure, not invented by Agamben but can be found earlier in Foucault's lectures in Paris. The idea of 'biopolitics' forms part of Foucault's overall critique of modern liberal political ideologies. His lectures, now published as *The Birth of Biopolitics* (2008) focused on the centrality of 'life' and how the modern liberal political ideologies began to think in terms of 'population' management. Agamben's theory of biopolitics can also be seen as a continuation of Heidegger's idea of inception, the idea that western thought follows a trajectory that is founded on the Greek notion of an originary *arche*.

Heidegger, technology and thinking

It is quite obvious that the modern state relies heavily on technology as a way of expanding its power. The COVID-19 global pandemic is probably one of the most disruptive events in recent history, and it is also certainly quite unexpected. In the face of such a disruptive event it is interesting to note how so many governments in the world are exclusively focused on technology as a way of solving problems. The pandemic saw the emergence of new technological devices and methods as a way to fight the virus. However, most of these are linked to surveillance, movement control and vaccines. Governments invested heavily in these new surveillance technologies in order to detect possible transmissions between people, in identification devices that control movement as well as in new vaccines to combat the virus. Technology dominates the current discourse in the fight against Covid. If we read the history of technology, however, we will discover that the use of new technologies is not without their side effects. Oftentimes many of these side effects are unexpected and harmful, and it takes some time before further refinements make them safe for use. The fact is that new technologies usually bring about 'unintended consequences'. That is, the new technological cures may solve the intended problem, but they can also contribute to the problem they are designed to solve, or give birth to new problems that were unforeseen. Many of these problems sometimes may even outweigh the benefits received. To be sure, recognizing the limitations of technology does not mean that we should stop using or developing new technologies altogether. The development and use of new technologies, with proper care for their unintended side effects can lead to the appearance of responsible technologies. The problem is not in adopting the technological frame of mind, and the solution is not in abandoning technology altogether. The problem is when this technological frame of mind becomes the only frame of mind. Heidegger famously observed that human beings as *dasein* are able to relate to the world using different frames of mind. They are 'open' to the world in a sense. Human beings can relate to the world in terms of *phronesis*, as in virtuous doing, and they can relate to the world in terms of *poesis*, by being open to its mysterious unveiling. This seems to have changed as human beings' relation to the world became more and more technological, in the sense of regarding everything as a mere *tool* to be used, and eventually the natural world came to be seen as a mere *resource* that is 'standing there' and waiting to be used and exploited by us, as mere 'standing reserve' (*Bestand*) (Heidegger 1977, 17). Thus, the history of the world may be seen as a journey from multiple valid ways of thinking towards one single way of thinking that. The later Heidegger would recommend a 'letting-be' (*Gelassenheit*) of this frame of mind in relation to technology (Heidegger 1966, 54). The word *Gelassenheit* was borrowed from Meister Eckhardt, a thirteenth-century German mystic and theologian and it suggests of an attitude of attentive care towards technology. There is no sense of trying to 'overcome' technology, as Heidegger would later realize, for this merely reinforces the metaphysics of technological thinking.

This analysis of the primordial influence of biopolitical thinking is valuable as it warns us of the expansion of power during this pandemic. However, there are a number of issues with this analysis. One of the first is how are we to effect this 'letting-be' in the first place? The act of 'stepping back' in relation to technology, which Heidegger recommends, seems to be reasonable but not very viable, we remember that *dasein* is already submerged in the middle of metaphysics and technological thinking. Second, even though such analyses warn us about the rise of biopolitics, this leaves us with very little in terms of what we *ought* to do, and what we *can* do in the face of the rise of biopolitics. From a Deleuzian perspective, even if we accept that the Greeks have influenced the development of our thinking, it remains contingent and not necessary. In the words of Deleuze and Guattari, this is expressed by Janae Sholtz: 'For Deleuze, it is not that the conjunction of the Greek territory and Western earth is wrong, but that to continue to return to this origin is reductive' (Sholtz 2015, 237). Third, from a Deleuzian perspective, as concepts are there to solve problems, it is not clear how the concept of biopolitics serves to solve problems. There is even an echo of messianism in Agamben's thought that, to use a Deleuzian-Spinozaic terminology, can only offer us passive knowledge but not active and immanent image-of-thought which empowers us to act for radical change in our present times.

Deleuze's theory of state

Deleuze, together with Guattari, offers us a theory of state that complements some of Agamben's most important insights on biopolitics. To begin with, we need to see that there are some similarities in the two theories. First, what they share in common is the idea that the state is not a concrete entity but something abstract. Deleuze regards the 'State-form' as an *abstract* model of power that is based on particular institutions and practices, which is yet somehow 'more than' these particular actualizations. The State is, according to Deleuze, not a concrete entity but an abstract machine that overcodes and regulates minute institutions and practices. In *Dialogues II* (1987) Deleuze states that 'the apparatus of the State is a concrete assemblage which realises the machine of overcoding of a society. This machine is not the State itself, but an abstract machine which organises the dominant utterances, feelings and established order of a society' (1987, 129). Second, both Deleuze and Guattari's analysis of the State and Agamben's theory of biopolitics also have in common in that they do not presume that the state is based on economic exchange. For Deleuze and Guattari, the State did not arise after production but in fact predates production. Deleuze and Guattari say: 'It is not the State that presupposes a mode of production; quite the opposite, it is the State that makes productions a "mode"' (1987, 429). For Deleuze and Guattari, there has always been the State and this is known as the *Urstaat*, an eternal State which comes into existence fully formed. Likewise, Agamben bases biopolitics on a foundational *arche* which can be found in Greek thought. Third, their theories also resonate with each other as they see the modern state-forms as being integrated with global capitalism. In *A Thousand Plateaus* (1987), Deleuze, together with Guattari, argues that the State may be seen as 'an apparatus of capture' with 'the power of appropriation' (1987, 437). What this means is that the State is the apparatus that codes economic flows and flows of production, organizing them into a mode. Agamben's theory of biopolitics also does not preclude the subterranean involvements that contemporary state-forms have with global capital. Fourth, in *A Thousand Plateaus* (1987) Deleuze, together with Guattari, writes that in modern times it makes no difference whether the State takes on an 'authoritarian', a 'socialist' or a 'liberal democratic' formation. As an abstract machine these different state-forms are all equivalent to each other insofar as they are political models that work with the aim of accumulating global capital. There is thus a sort of complementarity between First World democratic states and Third World dictatorships (Deleuze and Guattari 1987, 465). Agamben's theory of biopolitics is basically in agreement with this since the integration with global capitalism means that modern state forms, even though they may be legitimized on the basis of modern liberal democratic processes or economic success, actually work to maintain the global system of exploitation and repression on working citizens.

Although there are resonances between Deleuze and Guattari's analysis of the state and Agamben's idea of biopolitics, there are also important differences which need to be highlighted. First, Deleuze and Guattari's theory of the State goes beyond mere critique and focuses on the relationship between the State and thinking. Deleuze and Guattari's State does not legitimize itself without thinking. Deleuze is known for saying that thought is 'already in conformity with a model that it borrows from the State apparatus, and which defines for its goals and paths, conduits, channels, organs, an entire *organon*' (Deleuze and Guattari 1987, 374). An example of this form of thinking is none other than our usual understanding of rationality itself. Instead of seeing certain forms of thought as simply lending rational and moral authority to the State, Deleuze argues that rational and moral discourses themselves in fact form part of the assemblage of the State. These discourses do not simply provide conceptual justifications for the State; in reality, they are the immediate manifestations of the State form itself. The State is immanent in thought, giving it ground, logos – providing it with a model that defines its 'goal, paths, conduits, channels, organs' (Deleuze and Guattari 1987, 374). The State has penetrated and coded thought, in particular rational thought. It both depends on rational discourses for its legitimization and functioning while in turn making these discourses possible. Rational thought is State philosophy: 'Common sense, the unity of all the faculties at the centre of the Cogito, is the State consensus raised to the absolute' (Deleuze and Guattari 1987, 376). In Deleuze's analysis, this means that in order to free ourselves from the State, we have no other way to do so than by freeing thought from this moral and rational authoritarianism.

Second, while Deleuze and Guattari and Agamben would agree that the State is not something concrete but *abstract* it is also important to note that Deleuze and Guattari's critique is not exactly the same as an ideological critique. Despite Deleuze and Guattari's acknowledgement that they are 'Marxists', this is only in the sense that they engage in a critique of the state insofar as it is integrated with global capitalism in such a way that it leads to the oppression of the workers. They do not show an alignment with the traditional Marxist idea of class warfare and progress in stages. In *Anti-Oedipus* (1983), Deleuze and Guattari make it clear that they disagree with 'ideological critiques' of the State because they are overly focused on the *cognitive* aspect of social structures. An exclusive focus on the cognitive aspect of social structures can be problematic because it results in neglecting the *affective* aspect of social structures. While ideological critiques have some uses as they are focused on correcting the irrationality that pervades society, hoping to make them more 'rational', they do so with the assumption that people are innocent and simply being misled into accepting irrational beliefs and ideological constructs. Deleuze and Guattari's theory of the state is not just a political idea, it also dives deep into the people's desire and excavates the direct libidinal investments that they may have invested in their oppressive social structures. Deleuze and Guattari state:

> Reich is at his profoundest as a thinker when he refuses to accept ignorance or illusion on the part of the masses as an explanation of fascism, and demands an explanation that will take their desires into account, an explanation formulated in term of desire: no, the masses were not innocent dupes; at a certain point, under a certain set of conditions, they wanted fascism, and it is this perversion of the desire of the masses that needs to be accounted for (Deleuze and Guattari 1983, 29).

This obviously shows that Deleuze and Guattari do not agree with ideological critique because they simply assume that the source of oppression is cognitive, which can be solved by cognitive means. From the perspective of Deleuze and Guattari, the real source of oppression lies not in cognitive errors but in the people's perverse desires. Hence, Deleuze and Guattari remind us that our behaviour is:

> not a question of ideology. There is an unconscious libidinal investment of the social field that coexists, but does not necessarily coincide, with the preconscious investments, or with what the preconscious investments 'ought to be.' That is why, when subjects, individuals, or groups act manifestly counter to their class interests –when they rally to the interests and ideals of a class that their own objective situation should lead them to combat – it is not enough to say: they were fooled, the masses have been fooled. It is not an ideological problem, a problem of failing to recognize, or of being subject to, an illusion. It is a problem of desire, *and desire is part of the infrastructure* (Deleuze and Guattari 1983, 104; my emph.).

What is perverse about fascist desire is that it is a form of desire that desires its own repression. This is why Deleuze and Guattari insist that Reich is correct when he emphasizes the priority of psychic repression. To be sure, this does not mean that

Deleuze and Guattari are in complete agreement with Reich's theory. What they find problematic is that Reich reinstalls a distinction between rational social production and irrational fantasies; that is, Reich assumed that there was the old split between *desire* as irrational fantasy and *production* as rational reality, and so he failed to see how desire can also be productive, i.e. desiring-production. Thus, from Deleuze and Guattari's perspective, Reich's psychoanalytic view of desire remains negative and fails to grasp the positive potential of desire. Deleuze and Guattari state: 'But, since he had not sufficiently formulated the concept of desiring-production, he did not succeed in determining the insertion of desire into the economic infrastructure itself, the insertion of the drives into social production' (1983, 118–119). When we see desiring-production for what it is, we begin to see that in the current state-form it is those who are oppressed who possess the direct libidinal investment in the very system that oppresses them. Deleuze and Guattari say that '[d]esire of the most disadvantaged creature will invest with all its strength, irrespective of any economic understanding or lack of it, the capitalist social field as a whole' (1983, 229). This means that ideological critiques are inadequate as they are confined to the task of identifying and critiquing cognitive errors. Such critiques miss the most important component of unjust social systems, namely, desire, and so a reliance on them will be counterproductive.

Rhizomaic-thinking vs. State-thinking

For Deleuze the project of resisting the State-form begins with the recognition of State-thinking. State-thinking is based on a particular type of thinking called *aborescent* thinking. This refers to a conceptual model or an 'image' which predetermines the trajectory of thinking on a rational basis. Deleuze says: 'Now, there is no doubt that trees are planted in our heads: the tree of life, the tree of knowledge, etc. The whole world demands roots. Power is always arborescent' (1987, 25). This is like the root and tree system in that it assumes that there is a central unity, like the root and its trunk, from which is determined the growth of its 'branches'. Deleuze says:

> [T]rees are not a metaphor at all, but an image of thought, a functioning, a whole apparatus that is planted in thought in order to make it go in a straight line and produce the famous correct ideas. There are all kinds of characteristics in the tree: there is a point of origin, seed or centre; it is a binary machine or principle of dichotomy, with its perpetually divided and reproduced branchings, its points of arborescence (1987, 25).

The internalization of this form of thinking means that we are immediately trapped in such a way that our thinking must now unfold according to a dialectical fashion, and in a logic of binary division that is fundamentally opposed to difference and plurality (Deleuze 1987, 128).

Instead of this authoritarian model of thought, Deleuze proposes a *rhizomatic* form of thinking. A rhizomatic form of thinking avoids traditionally accepted unities and binary logic, instead, it seeks out multiplicities, pluralities and *becomings*. It is a form of non-authoritarian 'image' of thought that is based on the metaphor of grass which grows haphazardly and imperceptibly, as opposed to the orderly growth of the aborescent tree system. This rhizomatic thinking defies the very idea of a model or a tree and chooses instead a haphazard multiplicity of connections which is not dominated by a single centre or place, but is decentralized and plural. Such a thinking is opposed to the very idea of binary divisions and hierarchies, and is not governed by an unfolding, dialectical logic. It thus interrogates the abstractions that govern thought, which form the basis of various discourses of knowledge and rationality. In other words, rhizomatic thought is thought which defies Power by refusing to be limited by it.

Deleuze and Guattari's rhizomatic thinking has radical implications for political philosophy. While political philosophy is based on the traditional battle lines between the State and individual rational subjects, rhizomatic thought forms multiple connections between subjects, including connections with the State that it is 'opposing'. In *A Thousand Plateaus*, Deleuze and Guattari say: 'These lines always tie back to one another. That is why one can never posit a dualism or a dichotomy, even in the rudimentary form of the good and the bad' (1987, 9). The simple fact is that the dichotomy between the State and its subjects is an artificial one, and any resistance based on this dichotomy invariably reinforces State power. Therefore, Deleuze and Guattari see political theories that are based on rational critiques of the State, to be forms of thinking which actually reaffirm State power instead of resisting it. By viewing the State as fundamentally irrational, and their own critiques as rational, they are unable to recognize the simple fact that the State has already *captured* rational discourse itself. This means that the very act of subverting the State does not subvert it but actually affirms it. This means that if the State is to be overcome we must abandon the project of criticizing the State on a Rational basis, and try to invent new forms of politics which do not allow themselves to be captured by rationality. In *Dialogues II*, Deleuze reminds us that '[p]olitics is active experimentation, since we do not know in advance which way a line is going to turn' (1987, 137).

From such a Deleuzian framework, what might be a Deleuzian response to the rise of biopolitics? I believe that Deleuze had a highly *relational* concept of the state, in the sense that that from a Deleuzian perspective, the function of the state is not an absolute one but one which is in fact highly relative and contextual. While it is important to realize is that while there is an expansion of state power through technologies, these technologies are not necessarily fascist in themselves but can have liberating functions. While history has shown that technologies are controlled by the elites in society, in order to bolster and maintain the status quo, there is no reason why these technologies cannot be used to resist the elites themselves. A Deleuzian perspective towards biopolitical technologies would have to be a *creative* one and not one that is restricted to a negative critique of technology or biopolitics. Furthermore, even as we are stunned momentarily by the impact of the COVID-19 pandemic, there is no reason why we cannot see the pandemic as a moment in history in which people throughout the world are frozen in their tracks and begin to question what is really important in their lives, and what is not, and become committed to global and planetary causes. After all, Deleuze and Guattari remind us that for thinking to truly occur, it has to come 'from the outside'. The pandemic, if anything, constitutes precisely this outside that carries with it the potential for change. In Heideggerian language, the pandemic is *an Event* that breaks through the metaphysical world that that we have constructed for ourselves since the Greeks. In terms of resistance, has the pandemic also highlighted the importance of collective practices that actually improve the health of populations, including large-scale behaviour modifications, without a parallel expansion of forms of coercion and surveillance? I believe that the answer is yes.

The nature of technology is such that it is highly ambiguous, possessed of multiple potentials that simply cannot be reduced to their 'designed functions'. The law of 'unintended consequences' strikes both ways. To be sure, a designer of a specific technology may have a particular function in mind for that technology, but the technology may come to possess other functions that are unthought of by the designer. To think otherwise is to assume that technologies can only have the specific functions that the designers designed them for. This would be an absurd way of thinking. This is why even though philosophers should be wary of the rise of biopolitics via various technologies and medical mandates, we should not forget at the same time that these technologies afford a multiplicity of potentialities. Indeed, while it is true that the new technologies in surveillance and movement control can lead to the loss of privacy and even human rights, it is also important to note that these same technologies can be used to resist biopolitical control. Just to take one example, the increased access to knowledge, something unimaginable a generation before, makes possible collective sharing of information and decision processes that are based on mutual interests and understanding and not just on the authority of state-sanctioned 'experts'. Furthermore, we need to think of how new information technologies have enabled us to become more aware of global and planetary events and how they help us to see the interconnectedness of peoples and their environments. While the new technologies could generate fear and insecurities in the population, there is also a corresponding greater access to knowledge. They can help us question official narratives and ultimately make it clear that we need to have critical thinking. The frustration that accompanies the numbers may also not make us accept the official narrative but make us realize that the decisions of life and death cannot be left to inefficient governments and 'experts'. In some cases, these surveillance technologies can help us to connect globally and to organize new global movements that cut across narrow nationalistic confines.

The challenge to rhizomatic thinking lies in its immanence. In *What is Philosophy?* (1994) Deleuze and Guattari say that: 'Immanence is immanent only to itself and consequently captures everything, absorbs All-One, and leaves nothing remaining to which it could be immanent. In any case, whenever immanence is interpreted as immanent *to* Something, we can be sure that this Something reintroduces the transcendent' (1994, 45). From an immanent standpoint, the thinker asks 'given my existing powers, what are my capabilities, what are my capacities, and how can I come into active possession of my power so that I can live a fuller life?' Daniel W. Smith, in *Essays on Deleuze* (2012), has highlighted this point by saying that from this immanent perspective, ethics is a set of 'facilitative' rules that measure the extent to which we have lived a life of intensity (2012, 147). The challenge is in seeing how we are to engage in this form of thinking when it has no external references. Deleuze and Guattari recognize this when they say in *What Is Philosophy?* that the real task of philosophy is to address the question of how we can acquire an immanent consistency without losing the infinity into which thought plunges. Unlike science, which is able to provide chaos with simple and straightforward reference points that enable us to proceed, philosophy asks how we can have these reference points without losing the infinite. Deleuze and Guattari hold that the supreme task of philosophy may not be to think *the* plane of immanence but simply to show that it is there, as the base of all planes, and as such immanent to every plane. It is that which remains unthought – it is that which cannot be thought but which *must* be thought, and which was thought once, as Christ was incarnated once, to show the possibility of the impossible (Deleuze and Guattari 1994, 59). This can be framed in an ethical framework. Ian Buchanan has highlighted this when he says that one of the persistent problems in Deleuze studies is the question of 'what is the right thing to do?' He says 'there is nothing at all within Deleuze and Guattari's theory of desire that can tell us either how we should live or how we should treat others' (Buchanan 2011, 18). This does not mean that we should abandon such projects, but that we need to recognize that such projects are not straightforward but rather a task that needs to be constructed.

In short, the strength of Deleuze and Guattari's theory of politics is that it links up the formation of the state with desire, so any change in the state would require a shift in thinking and desire. However, as this requires transformation in thinking, a transformation which requires an outside that it does not in principle have access to, this means that it is structurally similar to Agamben's *messianic* reading of the state. In other words, even if we accept in principle that rhizomatic-thinking is better than state-thinking, how is it possible for Deleuze and Guattari's rhizomatic-thinking to replace state-thinking, when so many in society do not seem to have a strong desire or incentive for thinking in the first place? Instead, the dominant mode of thinking seems to be the sort of thinking that is directed by a desire for more power, control and surveillance. If anything, living in a state-dominated society also fosters an abrogation of individual responsibility, a lust for more authority and resentment for those who are different from us.

In other words, while both Heideggerian and Deleuzian inspired reflections would agree that we need to bring about a different way of thinking during this pandemic, there remains the issue of *how* we are to bring about this change. Now Deleuze and Heidegger are basically in agreement that we live in an age of unthinking. Heidegger is famous for his reflection on thinking (*Denken*) when he states in *What Is Called Thinking?* (1968) that 'what is most thought-provoking is that we are still not thinking' (1968, 4). Deleuze would also insist that in order to think we would need to confront the fact of stupidity in society. Indeed, Deleuze himself has suggested in *Nietzsche and Philosophy* that '[t]he use of philosophy is to *sadden* [*attrister*]. A philosophy that saddens no one, that annoys no one, is not a philosophy. It is useful for harming stupidity [bêtise], for turning stupidity into something shameful' (2002, 106). Second, in order to think we need to go beyond the discipline that is called philosophy. Heidegger insists that we need to go beyond the discipline of philosophy and to move towards what he calls 'thinking'. One way of doing this is by way of turning towards poetry. Following Heidegger, Deleuze states: 'An image of thought called philosophy has been formed historically and it effectively stops people from thinking' (Deleuze and Parnet 2002, 13). One way in which Deleuze 'democratized' thinking is by way of expanding the possibility of thinking by including the arts. One example of this is by way of his cinema books. Deleuze holds that cinema can 'arouse the thinker in you', unfolding involuntary thinking (1989, 279). Third, Heidegger has also argued that thinking is not a natural process and that it needs a struggle. Likewise, Deleuze argues that thinking does not come naturally but requires a degree of force from the outside. Deleuze holds that: 'What is essential is outside of thought, in what forces us to think' (2002, 95). The question remains as to what constitute this 'outside' that will force us to think.

Conclusion

The COVID-19 global pandemic certainly unveils the relationship between the modern state form and technological thinking. Agamben's theory of biopolitics helps us to understand how the state of exception may be extended in the name of a health-security regime but, not unlike Heidegger's analysis of modern technological and metaphysics, and his recommendation of 'letting-be' gives us the feeling that nothing can be done and that 'only a god can save us'. Deleuze's theory of state and state-thinking seem to give us a more insightful and practical concept by which we may peep into the mechanics of desire. The question remains, however, as to how is this radical shift in desire can become a possibility, when desire is always already implicated in state-thinking. In other words, where is this desire that replaces existing desires to arise from? The task of thinking is yet to be complete and maybe, just maybe, the rise of biopolitics in the midst of this COVID-19 global pandemic is 'the outside' that will force us to take up the task of thinking.

References

Agamben, Giorgio (1998), *Homo Sacer: Sovereign Power and Bare Life*, trans. D. Heller-Roazen, Stanford and California: Stanford University Press.

Agamben, Giorgio (2000), *Means without Ends: Notes on Politics*, trans. V. Binetti and C. Casarino, London and Minneapolis: University of Minnesota Press.

Agamben, Giorgio (2005), *State of Exception*, trans. K. Attell, Chicago and London: University of Chicago Press.

Agamben, Giorgio (2020), 'The Invention of an Epidemic' (published in Italian on *Quodlibet*, https://www.quodlibet.it/giorgio-agamben-l-invenzione-di-un-epidemia).

Agamben, Giorgio (2021), *Where Are We Now? The Epidemic as Politics*, trans. V. Dani, London: Eris.

Buchanan, Ian (2011), 'Desire and Ethics', *Deleuze Studies Vol. 5*, Edinburgh: Edinburgh University Press, pp. 7–20.

Deleuze, Gilles (1987), *Dialogues II*, trans. H. Tomlinson, New York: Columbia University Press.

Deleuze, Gilles (1989), *Cinema 2: Time-Image*, trans. H. Tomlinson and R. Galeta, London: Athlone Press.

Deleuze, Gilles (2002), *Nietzsche and Philosophy*, trans. H. Tomlinson, London: Continuum.
Deleuze, Gilles and Felix Guattari (1983), *Anti-Oedipus: Capitalism and Schizophrenia*, Minneapolis: University of Minnesota Press.
Deleuze, Gilles and Felix Guattari (1987), *A Thousand Plateaus: Capitalism & Schizophrenia*, trans. B. Massumi, Minneapolis: University of Minnesota Press.
Deleuze, Gilles and Felix Guattari (1994), *What Is Philosophy?* trans. H. Tomlinson and G. Burchell, New York: Columbia University Press.
Deleuze, Gilles and Claire Parnet (2002), *Dialogues II*, trans. H. Tomlinson, B. Habberjam, E. Albert, London: Continuum.
Foucault, Michel (2008), *The Birth of Biopolitics: Lectures at the College De France 1978–1979*, edited by M. Senelart, trans. G. Burchell, London: Palgrave.
Heidegger, Martin (1966) *Discourse on Thinking: A Translation of Gelassenheit* (trans. J. M. Anderson and E. H. Freund). New York: Harper & Row.
Heidegger, Martin (1968), *What Is Called Thinking?* trans. J. Glenn Gray, New York: Harper.
Heidegger, Martin (1977), *The Question Concerning Technology and Other Essays*, trans. W. Lovitt, New York: Harper Collins.
Sholtz, Janae (2015), *The Invention of a People: Heidegger and Deleuze on Art and the Political*, Edinburgh: Edinburgh University Press.
Smith, Daniel W. (2012), *Essays on Deleuze*, Edinburgh, Edinburgh University Press.

5

Post-Covid Communities: A Schizoanalysis of Immanent Engagements

Janae Sholtz

Covid has brought the realities of our material continuity and our unavoidable proximities to light in ways that are challenging the efficacy of traditional socio-political ideals of individualism and autonomy. Moreover, the stark reality that community is primarily regarded in economic rather than spiritual or ethical terms lies at the base of the problematic responses that we have seen (this is especially true from my US perspective). For a post-Covid future to be anything but dystopian, the parameters of community and individuality will need to be rethought and a deeper awareness of our immanent immersive engagements fostered. There are resources both in Deleuzian philosophy and posthumanism and new materialist feminisms that can be marshalled for imagining such post-Covid communities. I will argue that the new materialist view of the interconnectedness of matter (where materiality as such is understood as intra-active and entangled) is a crucially necessary shift in mindset – the obvious benefit is providing a basis and rationale for our moving beyond the rampant individualism that has evidenced itself – at least in the US response. Post-Covid futures require the re-evaluation of the nature of ethical relationships, notions of subjectivity, and political imperatives in a post-Covid world. In what follows, I will address the following three issues: 1) The 'I' in a post-Covid era; 2) Social responsibilities of the citizens in the Covid pandemic; 3) The post-covid era and alternative futures.

The 'I', post-Covid

If Covid has revealed anything to me, it is that we need a paradigm shift with respect to how we understand the 'I' (and I acknowledge that I speak from a particular location – as an American in the United States where what we have seen is an utter refusal to give up our rampant individualism, a doubling down on individual rights over the good of the community, and where any discussion of 'institutions or collective goods' decisions are being driven by neo-liberal concern for economic prosperity – which is itself based on the liberal paradigm of self-interest). It is not enough to pose more community-mindedness or to be more generous, more empathetic, without addressing the deep-seated belief in metaphysical individualism that supports our insistence on the individual as the primary figure of ethical concern.

According to Félix Guattari, the posthuman predicament (and one could equally say, our post-Covid predicament) calls for a new virtual social ecology, in which we must think of the subject, or subjectivities, transversally – breaking down barriers between the ecologies of environment, the social nexus and the psyche. In other words, we must think of the subject as 'ontologically polyvocal'. This poses new challenges for philosophy – to reach across disciplinary boundaries to consider the ways that new developments in the sciences for instance have changed our understanding of the nature of matter, the bios, the environment and our relation to it. This is exactly what new materialist feminists like Rosi Braidotti, Karen Barad, Donna Haraway and Elizabeth Grosz, in different respects obviously, have proposed. By incorporating the realizations of quantum physics, biochemistry and Darwinian evolution, to name a few of the interdisciplinary areas of inquiry, their main philosophical point is that matter has been historically devalued and seen as inert, passive and deprioritized in relation to all things related to mind and thought and, thus, 'thinking anew about the fundamental structure of matter [will have] far-reaching normative and existential implications' (Coole and Frost 2010, 5).

There are two main points with regard to matter mattering: First, new materialists insist upon on the dynamism (or agency) of matter as the constitutive force of the objects/assemblages that arise, rather than viewing matter as mediated or acted upon by an agent or the external force of culture or history and explain causation or the becoming of matter as processes of agential forces. They insist on the role of 'an excess, force, vitality, relationality, or difference that renders matter active, self-creative, productive, unpredictable' (Coole and Frost 2010, 9). This also impacts their understanding of the role of matter and nonhuman actors in the production of knowledge and in the production of subjectivities. Matter and bodies are not only formed by the forces of language, culture and politics but are also formative – which means that our 'selves' are not just formed through human actions, between individual subjects, but that we are part of intra-actions with the very 'objects' that our reliance on individualism have carved out.

This is exemplified by Covid on multiple levels, and such an understanding is crucial to bypass the politicization that we have seen, particularly here in the United States. A virus has a life and vivacity of its own; it is immune to linguistic structures, rhetorical posturing, political manoeuvring. Yet our obliviousness to the vitality or agency of matter, which could very well be a consequence of the deeply embedded philosophical view of the passivity and inertness of matter, is explanation for our unwillingness to cede space and control or to address the issue of our commonality in the face of this pandemic: we literally share the same space, are connected by breath, air, viral and chemical exchanges, and we must not address the post-Covid world in terms of our individual actions, desires or interests, as if we were autonomous little nodules of freedom. Second, this reconceptualization of matter leads to a reconfiguration of metaphysical priority and understanding. New materialists realize that the subject/object division indicative of metaphysical individualism obscures the real relations and imbrication of entities with milieus of materiality and obscures the ontological level of incessant transformation and process. Donna Haraway, for instance, holds that beings do not pre-exist their 'relatings' (process ontology); Karen Barad (2007) develops the term intra-actions to indicate that entities are not distinct prior to the relation of components but rather emerge from within; and Stacy Alaimo (2010) challenges the assumption of bodily boundaries with the concept of trans-corporeality: '*Trans* indicates movement across different sites, trans-corporeality also opens up a mobile space that acknowledges the often unpredictable and unwanted actions of human bodies, nonhuman creatures, ecological systems, chemical agents, and other actors' (Alaimo 2010, 2). Moreover, they agree that relations do not operate by a linear causal model but through networks, assemblages, focusing on the materiality of these assemblages as constitutive of the objects that arise rather than matter as mediated or acted upon by an agent or the external force of culture or history. This is essential to Barad's concept of agential realism and Bennet's vibrant matter (2010): 'Objects always exist in dynamic "assemblages" and connections that affect what they are and how they behave. Accordingly, it does not make sense to conceive of an object as a bounded and distinct thing – as if it existed in isolation from other objects and humans' (Bennett 2004, 365). New materialists, therefore, provide an important backdrop for assessing global, non-localizable and fluid phenomena, as well as providing us with a new theoretical vantage point on who and what are 'subjects', that decentralizes the priority of purely human relations and, rather, understands subjectivity as a set of processes that include multiple components and partners – human, animal and organic. Rosi Braidotti, for instance, wants to enlarge the frame and scope of subjectivity along the transversal lines of post-anthropocentric relations. Human subjectivity would be re-defined as an expanded relational self, which includes nonhuman others, but it also allows us to open up (and acknowledge) the virtual forces of Life.

Why is this helpful? First, to navigate a post-Covid world, the materialist account of the vitality of matter and our 'selves' as relationally embedded in a series of intra-actions may help us understand the event that is happening to us. Covid, as a viral living matter, doesn't know boundaries – either geographically or bodily – and it certainly doesn't play political favourites or respect rights. Simply put, intra-action is a better way of understanding our situatedness with respect to Covid. We are dealing with a new reality where we had better begin to respect the manner in which we are ineluctably bound to (in fact formed through) our environments and various materialities. Second, in rejecting the longstanding dogma of metaphysical individualism, we may find room for thinking of new forms of sociality and community which incorporate the idea of open-ness, diversity of typologies, and privilege relations and encounters over rights and self-interest. Third, as Angela Merkel said over the summer while addressing a plenary session at the European Parliament in Brussels on 8 July 2020, Covid 'highlights the limits of fact-denying populism'. This seems to be so across the world, but, unfortunately, not in the United States. Not only is philosophy needed more than ever to lay out the parameters of truth versus lie, but as a philosophical practice that acknowledges and incorporates the facts of science.

Social responsibilities of citizens in the pandemic

I will begin to address the issue of responsibility with a negative characterization, in terms of what we lack as a society. I think in doing so, we may begin to derive a sense of the third theme of this chapter: post-Covid alternative futures. First, there is a marked lack of imagination involved in our present reality, which manifests in the largescale inability to imagine from another's point of view and the inability to imagine different futures. Second, our society lacks empathy, a close relation to the lack of ability to imagine another's point of view, but one which extends even further by morphing into perverse cruelty and delight at the suffering of others. The unfortunate fact in the United States is that this has become almost a national character trait – ubiquitous and all-encompassing – because it has been baked into the mainstream American psyche through the logics of misogyny and racism, which require and encourage both dehumanizing women and minorities and punishment for not adhering to the rules of the ruling class. Third, we lack emplaced awareness, a reality which has been fostered philosophically by the separation of mind and body, politically through the cult of individualism, and culturally through the historical practices of geographical segregation and contemporary isolation of virtual spaces/online cultures that allow for a kind of aggression through anonymity, which then spills over into material forms of violence. I am thinking of the way that the Incel movement (see Williams 2018) festered and developed the psyche of several young men who then took guns and indiscriminately slaughtered women, as women *in general* became emblems of all that was 'wrong' with their lives, or how the dark web has fomented white supremacy and been linked to the manifestos of several actual mass murders recently in the United States. Lack of emplaced awareness has consequences, anaesthetizing us to certain material realities, and especially differential material realities.

What do we need to do in light of these 'lacks' – i.e. what are the social responsibilities of the citizens in a Covid pandemic? There are several suggestions that either directly derive from or correlate with what I have said about new materialism. The following are drawn from these new materialist frameworks: 1) reconceptualizing the political in terms of encounters and involvedness, rather than liberties and rights; 2) reconsidering our modes of encountering 'others' (human and more-than-human); 3) prioritizing understanding relationships between the natural, human and nonhuman; inseparability of human processes from biochemical and physical; 4) developing an awareness for nonhuman vitality as a kind of perceptual openness; 5) focusing on epistemological limits and limits of human control.

The last point concerning epistemological limits is especially important to counteract the fact that we seem to be suffering in the United States from collective Dunning-Krueger, where those with the least knowledge present themselves as experts or the most knowledgeable (Trump) and literally denigrate and reject expert opinion (like the shameful vilification of Dr Anthony Fauci, the Director of the U.S. National Institute of Allergy and Infectious Diseases). This effect has spread like a collective neurosis, through the rank and file of the political right, and continues to spread through the wanton relativization of information vis-à-vis the vilification of critical new reporting and elevation of the cult of personality over content. New materialists ground the concept of epistemological humility on an ontological framework of openness and indeterminacy, the acknowledgement of which results from the ineluctable fact of our partial knowledge. The acknowledgement of the impossibility of complete knowledge – even as a goal – could really open up dialogue about our need for caution with regard to epistemic imperialism and arrogance, generating more empathetic connections and combatting forms of supremacy.

Diverging from the new materialist model

To varying degrees, new materialists accept some version of ontological immanence, which leads to a posthuman ethic, such that all entities are on equal ontological footing and no entity, whether artificial or natural, symbolic or physical, possesses greater ontological dignity than other objects. This is the cornerstone of the critique of anthropocentricism and posthuman turn – there is no privilege given to human/world relation as a form of metaphysical relation different in kind from other relations between objects. Thus, new materialism tends towards an ethico-political perspective of nonprivileged, nonhierarchical interactions (Braidotti's zoe-centred egalitarianism, 2013, 95) and which, according to one commentator, unfortunately results in a kind of 'ontological pacifism' (van Ingen 2016). There have been many critiques of this particular kind of universalization with respect to the political sphere. Robin James makes the salient point that focusing on the ontological universality of agency obscures the political question of the nonuniversality of personhood in her book, *The Sonic Episteme* (2019), and Juanita Sundberg amplifies this criticism, claiming that posthumanism 'tends to reproduce colonial ways of knowing and being by enacting universalizing claims' (2014, 33). We are faced with a situation which mirrors late twentieth-century critiques by U.S Third World feminist, Chela Sandoval (2000), and post-colonial thinkers such as Kwame Anthony Appiah (1991), of postmodernism and poststructuralism's creation of universalizing models that extract and abstract concepts of resistance and disruption in ways that occlude the real lived experience of the oppressed and source of said concepts. Both cases reveal the problem inherent to imposing abstract, theoretical models on the realm of ethics and politics, which renders attempts to acknowledge the discontinuities in experience moot under the guise of conceptual homogeneity or, in this case, ontological univocity. It is noteworthy that some of the most powerful critiques of the shift in ethics towards vital materialism often invoke a critical race perspective, calling attention to the homogenizing consequences of new materialist and posthumanist discourses of zoe-centred interconnectivity. Axelle Karera's (2019) article, 'Blackness and the Pitfalls of the Anthorpocene' is a brilliant exposition of the interventions of critical race theorists who profess scepticism with regard to the enthusiastic embrace of the new materialist/posthumanist zoe-centred approach (such as Leong 2016, Jackson 2015), and she is crystal clear with regard to the political stakes:

> [The] respective ethical and critical prescriptions of posthumanism [and new materialisms] sidestep an engaged account of social antagonisms, and more specifically those enacted along racial lines. Instead, these are smoothed over and

> displaced in the name of an ethics of futurity grounded on a deeply naturalized variation of relationality –namely that all beings, insofar as they are earthly at least, are fundamentally interconnected (Karera 2019, 43).

The insistence on attending to 'racial culpability' (Karera 2019, 44) and the discontinuities that exist in the socius because of the brutalities of racism is particularly important in assessing our social responsibilities during and after Covid – as mortality rates among minorities soar disproportionately, access to healthcare is particularly problematic for marginalized populations, and the administrative policies that force people back to work and insist upon school openings affect black populations in particular because of economic disparities which have resulted from decades of engineered dispossession and wealth theft. While the intent may be to foster a more equitable and nonhierarchical vision of inter-species relations and interactions, as Karera forcefully argues, the 'Anthropocene discourses, the "posthuman," the concept of life, and "relationality" are unequipped to account for the ongoing and brutal victimization of black people' (2019, 47). The various ways that personhood is conferred or not conferred due to oppression and racism in our country matter.

US third world feminists and so many women of color feminists have long argued that the shared political and social sphere does not mean that the space within which we are immersed, no matter how relationally, is shared equally or experienced in the same way – advocating for an intersectional politics that acknowledges ways that intersecting forms of oppression constrict and determine social identities. New materialists will insist that the particularity of embodiment, spatiality and situatedness with respect to power and oppression have to be considered, while maintaining that these discussions necessarily include attention to the relational milieus shared between corporeal entities, whether animal, vegetal or microbial; although there are some new materialists who do recognize that there is a lack of accommodation for issues of race and marginalization: 'we argue that race and the very processes through which racialized bodies come to matter (in both senses of the word) still have to be considered as areas that are underrepresented in many new materialist approaches' (Hinton et al. 2015, 1).

New materialists have come out rather forcefully against identity politics, and, unfortunately, this seems to have contributed to another species of the erasure of blackness, or, at least, that seems to be one of its casualties. The critique from poststructuralist philosophy and new materialists alike is that focusing on identities detracts from the underlying forces and conditions that are pre-personal, or nonhuman, subjectivity just solidifies a philosophical construct of the totality of self that erroneously places control in individuals and leads to exclusionary practices and the idea of mastery of nature and others. One of the key features of new materialist ontology is the insistence on the priority of relations over entities, that events are formed through intra-actions (assemblages). Barad explicitly contrasts her approach with that of *intersectionality*, which is an essential tool of feminist analysis of political oppression and difference. She views intersectionality as paradigmatic of feminist analysis associated with the cultural or linguistic turn (which new materialists are acting against). Thus, we see that between new materialist feminism and its supposed rivals or predecessor views, there is a rift. She claims that intersectionality has been developed as a 'mutually perpendicular set of axes of identification' (Barad 2001: 98) rather than iterative intra-actions through which a dynamic spatio-temporal scene is produced. Therefore, intersectional analysis remains at the level of mere opposition of already formed identities and identifies categories that become detached from a material foundation – i.e. identity politics – which become something of a lightning rod for criticism in the United States.

It seems to me that not only does new materialist' ontological immanence make it difficult to draw political distinctions, but their position against identity politics puts them at odds with intersectional feminists wanting to draw real distinctions concerning oppression and racism. In the United States, identity politics has become anathema to the left and right, and I fear that all discussions of identity or identities have become bound up in a reductive discourse. Ijeoma Oluo explains that criticizing identity politics has become the explanation *du jour* for why the left is divided – focusing too much on the needs and interests of particular 'identities', to the detriment of focus systemic economic issues that affect 'everyone' (2019, 8–9). Of course, on the right, it's more blatant – identity politics is just a bunch of whining social justice warriors complaining about their plights, which are largely mythic or their own fault anyway. Disciplines that are associated with certain 'identities', women's studies, African American studies, gender studies, are pejoratively referred to as 'grievance studies', to imply that discussions and focus on these groups are just reservoirs of whining rather than serious disciplines devoted to analysing and exposing deeply rooted power structures of oppression.

I have been guilty of miming this critique as well, and it comes with humility to say that I got it wrong. The version of identity politics that is touted is a caricature of the reason identity remains important to consider in political frameworks. The version of identity politics that seems to underlie these critiques is premised on an assumption that identity politics is just a 'mickey mouse' refrain of me, me, me. The problem seems to be the conflation of identity politics with individualism. Those espousing the importance of categories/identities are operating with a much more nuanced understanding of the function of identity in our society.

That the *perception* of identities is often ideological *is* the point. The identities of blackness, trans-ness, Hispanic, immigrant and myriad other minoritized positions in our (US) society are often associated with a constellation of assumptions, biases, negative connotations which create real conditions of oppression and injustice for people who 'fit' those categories, and these constructs, made of immaterial ideas, as well as institutional practices, laws and rules actually do foreground and shape material conditions and opportunities for creating relations. That is why we can't 'do away' with identity politics. It is not that identity is ontologically primary or even 'true' but that, regardless of these philosophical critiques, identity politics operates nonetheless. Some say that arguing along the lines of identity merely replicates and solidifies the fallacy of metaphysical individualism. But, in the spirit of Speaker Pelosi's usage of the phrase to counter the narrative that Democrats have focused too much energy on the idealistic goal of impeaching Trump to attend to their responsibilities to protecting citizens from Covid, we should be able to walk and chew gum at the same time. We can have a multi-pronged approach in how we analyse social formations *and* ontological forces, the accretions of historical, political oppressions and our immanent intra-relatedness. Even Gilles Deleuze, whom new materialists utilize in their full-throated dismissals of identity, recognizes that forces operate through self-ascribed, conscious interests (that are formulated along class lines, race lines, lines of identification) *and* unconscious lines of impersonal forces, affects and materialities – both the corporeal and the incorporeal.

Recognizing that identities are a conglomeration of associated affects and unconscious forces doesn't negate the reality of these perceptions. There is a reality of being black in America – unfortunately the experiences that accrue to that identity are often palpably brutal; they are immediate, well entrenched and overtly indiscriminate to 'personal or individual identity'. The social construct of identity is what identity politics is critiquing – so, ironically, identity politics (done in a sophisticated, critical manner) is the place where we attempt to deconstruct and eradicate the real effects of ideologies of identity, while building more positive communities. In other words, I don't think that identity politics (or intersectionality) works in the way that is being touted. Speaking about the systematic constraints that accrue to identities is not the solidification of an essentialized identity. Drawing from Donna Haraway's work (2008), Peta Hinton acknowledges that 'who speaks' is always, and necessarily, 'a community' (2014: 108).

So, while I find much in new materialism to admire – the alliance of philosophy and science to combat the hostility towards fact that has tainted both our administrative response and the public perception of the virus (i.e. refusal to wear masks, denial of the virus as a hoax), and the critique of the pernicious metaphysical individualism that has supported the egregious forms of atomistic self-interest and disproportionate focus on individual rights and liberty over public goods, like health and wellbeing – it is not a panacea for what ails us and cannot be the sole basis of a post-Covid future.

We need a way of thinking transversal relations, which attune us to how our 'selves' are formed and generated through immersive intra-actions, *along with* intersectional approaches that directly confront systems of oppression. Barad, and other new materialists, gravitate towards the transversal nature of the assemblage because it suggests the priority of relationality over identity, the *passage between* as a kind of becoming rather than merely an opposition of identities. In this respect (relationality), there are similarities between Barad's intra-action and Deleuze and Guattari's development of assemblages as interconnected relations, but this is also one of the places where the translation of Deleuzian concepts into the new materialist context fails to account for significant features that are important for critical analysis.

For Deleuze, assemblages are composed of co-constitutive and intra-active elements, but they do not all exist on the same level. Precisely the interests *and* desires of individuals and groups in society have to be addressed, accounted for, and examined for their quasi-causal impact, which Deleuze and Guattari identify as occupying two distinct levels – the molar and the molecular. Transversality, in Deleuze and Guattari, is more nuanced in that considerations of molarity (identity) and the molecular (preconscious flows, material flows, desires) that come into play are constituted as much by discontinuities – stops, breaks and gaps – as continuity. In *Anti-Oedipus*, Deleuze and Guattari (1983) emphasize that it is the cuts and breaks in machinic desire that are the motor of production. Analysing the relations between these fluctuating elements and how they produce singular events is the crux of schizoanalytic practice. The cartographies that accompany the diagnosis of parameters of interest and flows of desire can be very powerful tools in analysing the entire space of an encounter, the texture of an event.

As a mode of analysis, I propose the coupling of Deleuzian transversality and intersectionality, what I have elsewhere called "intersectional transversality" (see Sholtz 2019). This approach at once demands greater attunement to bodies and milieus, as well as insisting on rigorous socio-economic (anti-capitalist) analysis – with emphasis on the necessity of in-corporating theory (anchoring it in the specific lived experience of the marginalized), which is what I think must happen to produce post-Covid, ethical alternative futures.

Post-Covid era and alternative futures

Intersectional transversality would be a genealogical account that addresses spatio-temporal coordinates, unconscious investments of desire in relations which do not remain solely grounded between human beings, while simultaneously considering the operation of molar traits within the given social field that produce social identities. This provides the possibility for the disarticulation of subjectivity from these axes of identity, for loosening and rupturing molar boundaries in order to free movements of desire from certain pathways so that other unforeseen connections can be made, while remaining sensitive to the lessons of intersectional, third world and decolonial feminisms concerning the occlusion of the marginalized and tendencies towards abstraction reflected in much of the canonical philosophy of the West. It is to analyse the processes of desiring and unconscious investment at the juncture of *particular and historical* social formations. Intersectional transversality breaks with the emphasis on universal standards of individuality, through emphasis on an experience of locality and also by emphasizing transversal connections between heterogeneous types of formations – which means we can draw distinctions between entities in a way that satisfies a political agenda.

And, finally, intersectional transversality require a pedagogy of liminality: a *pedagogy of liminality* would involve tracing the limits that exist as social investments of desire and finding the contours of the different social assemblages and contexts, exploring these lines and contours by rejecting unidirectional linearity, finding ways that we can change the situations through different connections. Limits are also meeting places, points of connection. A pedagogy of liminality requires learning to trace those lines and meetings points, and, rather than eliminating paths, placing ourselves in these spaces. This could help engender new understanding of spatiality, which suggests the following: 1) the need for a careful process of diagramming of boundaries which eschews linear causality, and addresses the greater complexity of relational existence; 2) the need to resist rampant individualism and imposing our interests or viewpoints on others and the world, as a kind of ecological and political humility and resistance to androcentricism; 3) engendering new affective attunement – what I have called a *revolutionary form of loving* as a *differential spatial sensibility* (see Sholtz 2022).

Loving and political awareness

Loving is not merely a relation between subjects, but could be a relation to whole milieus, or environments. Simply put, it is not just *who* we love (identify with, form communities with) but *how* we love that is crucial. Love is a way of being in the world. Love as an intra-active milieu is an infinite process of learning/transformation through conjugation with otherness. This is an ecological, posthumanist approach to loving: to be in-formed (fully embodied and immanent) by our material engagements – *incorporated*. It expands the realm of love, invites our reconceptualization of the erotic, as an exploration of potentials of our whole bodies in congress with their environments, as intermingled with, tantalized and provoked by a plentitude of sensorial, material encounters, necessitating that we open ourselves, in thought and action, to the unfamiliar, the unknown and the other-worldly, as an interwoven dance of differences, pushing us beyond the concretizations of those worlds which may in fact inhibit us – political, socially, ethically and creatively, indicating a new capacity for intersubjective relation, one which gravitates toward singularity and undoes individualistic prerogatives that limit our abilities to engage with one another. Through 'infinite engagement with the otherness of our immanent and fluid relations to each other and the world' (Sholtz and Carr 2018: 461), we widen our understanding of what ethical loving and relations should be (and community for that matter). When we shift to the understanding of selves, as spatial cartographies, always dynamically involved with milieus, what Guattari calls existential territories, such a recognition lends itself to 'create new systems of valorization, a new taste for life, a new gentleness between the sexes, generations, ethnic groups, races' (1995, 92).

Revolutionary love is a revelation of our situatedness, and the love necessary to cede space to those whose versions of reality have been ignored or, worse, smothered. Granting this, it remains for many of us to embody that space differently, directing our awareness of the forces, affects and relations at play by sensitivity to that which is occluded. I want to suggest that we acknowledge the practice of 'holding space' as a way of ethically embodying space. Holding space has its origins in yoga and is a way of silencing one's ego and ceding space and time to the other – it is an intimate recognition of differential struggles, needs and obstacles to survival. It is meant to draw attention to the impositions, privilege or appropriations enacted by those of us who blithely occupy a form of dominant space on those who don't. It requires a stark assessment of one's privilege and position. In this respect, love as spatial awareness also acknowledges that many in our society (and world) have not had the luxury of occupying space freely or without threat. As I interpret Deleuze's own call for the minor-ization of philosophy, we prioritize the voices of the oppressed, the marginalized, and this goes for theory as well as the more literal, political spaces. We must read and elevate the discussions and bodies of work of critical race theorists, Black feminists, indigenous activists and thinkers, not ignore them or place them on some side of an imaginary divide (cartography) convenient for progressing certain narratives of theoretical inventiveness and superiority.

This is an alternative future in which we foster our attunement to material differences, while recognizing the contribution of those whose differential consciousness gives special purchase on our social situation. It is both posthuman and political intimacy, the vision of which becomes possible by aligning the rich histories of feminism, with their absolute insistence on elevating the voices and experiences of the politically disenfranchised and the conceptual framework of resistance and liberation culled from Deleuze and Guattari as well as new materialist ontology.

References

Alaimo, Stacy. 2010. *Bodily Natures*. Bloomington: Indiana University Press.

Appiah, Kwame Anthony. Winter 1991. 'Is the Post- in Postmodernism the Post- in Post- colonial?' *Critical Inquiry*. 17/2: 336–357.

Barad, Karen. 2001. 'Reconfiguring Space/Time Matter' in ed. Marianne De Koven. *Feminist Locations: Global and Local, Theory and Practice*. Brunswick, New Jersey: Rutgers University Press.

Barad, Karen. 2007. *Meeting the Universe Halfway, Quantum Physics and the Entanglement of Matter and Meaning*. Durham, North Carolina: Duke University Press.

Bennett, Jane. June 2004. 'The Force of Things: Steps towards and Ecology of Matter'. *Political Theory* 32.3: 347–372.

Bennet, Jane. 2010. *Vibrant Matter, A Political Ecology of Things*. Durham, North Carolina: Duke University Press.

Braidotti, Rosi. 2013. *The Posthuman*. Cambridge: Polity Press.

Coole, Diana and Samantha Frost. 2010. *New Materialisms Ontology, Agency, and Politics*. Durham, North Carolina: Duke University Press.

Deleuze, Gilles and Felix Guattari. 1983. *Anti-Oedipus: Capitalism and Schizophrenia*. Minneapolis: University of Minnesota Press.

Guattari, Félix. 1995. *Chaosmosis: An Ethico-Aesthetic Paradigm*, trans. Paul Bains and Julian Pefanis. Bloomington: Indiana University Press.

Haraway, Donna. 2008. 'Situated Knowledges: The Science Question in Feminism and The Privilege of Partial Perspective', *Feminist Studies* 14.3: 575–599.

Hinton, Peta. 2014. '"Situated Knowledges" and New Materialism(s): Rethinking a Politics of Location', *Women: A Cultural Review* 25.1: 99–113.

Hinton, Peta and Tara Mehrabi, Josef Barla. 2015. 'New Materialisms/New Colonialisms'. Åbo Akademi University, Finland: unpublished manuscript.

Jackson, Zakiyyah Iman. June 2015. 'Outer World: The Persistence of Race in the Movement "Beyond the Human"' *GLQ: A Journal of Gay and Lesbian Studies*, 21.2/3: 215–246.

James, Robin. 2019. *The Sonic Episteme: Acoustic Resonance, Neoliberalism, and Biopolitics*. Durham, North Caroline: Duke University Press.

Karera, Axelle. 2019. 'Blackness and the Pitfalls of the Anthropocene', *Critical Philosophy of Race*. 7.1: 32–56.

Leong, Diana. September 2016. 'The Mattering of Black Lives: Octavia Butler's Hyperempathy and the Promise of the New Materialism', *Catalyst Feminism Theory Technoscience*. 2.2: 1–35.

Oluo, Ijeoma. 2019. *So You Want to Talk about Race*. New York: Seal Press.

Sandoval, Chela. 2000. *The Methodology of the Oppressed*. Minnesota: University of Minnesota Press.

Sholtz, Janae. 2019. "Schizoanalysis and the Deterritorializations of Transnational Feminism," *Deleuze and the Schizoanalysis of Feminism*, Eds. J. Sholtz and C. L. Carr (London: Bloomsbury Press).

Sholtz, Janae. 2022. "Desire, Delirium, and Revolutionary Love: Deleuzian Feminist Possibilities," *Special Issue: Current French Philosophy in Difficult Times, Philosophies*, 7: 1-23.

Sholtz, Janae and Cheri Lynne Carr. Nov 2018. 'Infinite Eros'. Special Issue: *Infinite Eros: Deleuze, Guattari and Feminist Couplings* in *Deleuze and Guattari Studies*. 12.4: 455–465.

Sundberg, Juanita. January 2014. 'Decolonizing Posthumanist Geographies', *Cultural Geographies: Indigeneity and Ontology*. 21.1: 33–47.

Van Ingen, Michiel. August 2016. 'Beyond the Nature/Culture Divide? The Contradictions of Rosi Braidotti's *The Posthuman*', *Journal of Critical Realism*. 15: 530–542.

Williams, Zoe. 2018. 'Raw Hatred: Why the "Incel" Movement Targets and Terrorises Women'. *The Guardian*, https://www.theguardian.com/world/2018/apr/25/raw-hatred-why-incel-movement-targets-terrorises-women (retrieved 4 September 2020).

6

The Limits of Perception: Knights of Narcotics, Nonhuman Aesthetics and the Psychedelic Revival

Patricia Pisters

Introduction: Deleuze and Guattari and the psychedelic revival

And then the world came to a standstill. Since the beginning of the global COVID-19 pandemic in early 2020, habitual actions and ways of moving around and about have been interrupted, as sensori-motor schemes have been broken by lockdowns and curfews, by decelerated flows of transportation of people and goods, and by unconventional government measurements of different sorts and degrees. On a collective level, this interruption of our automatic behaviour resonates with Henri Bergson's philosophy of action in relation to perception in *Matter and Memory*. At the end of the nineteenth century, Bergson argued that, depending on the ability to move into sensori-motor action or the inability of habitual movement caused by any kind of sickness or disturbance, we enter into different 'tones' of psychic life. What is commonly held to be a disease or disorder of the psychic life, Bergson sees more positively as 'an unloosing or a breaking of the tie which binds psychic life to its motor accompaniment', which he considers as the 'mind striving to transcend the conditions of useful action and to come back to itself as to a pure creative energy' (Bergson 1991, 15).

While there is no direct causal link between the COVID-19 pandemic and the so-called psychedelic renaissance that has emerged since the early twenty-first century, it seems that both contemporary phenomena relate to finding what Bergson saw as a different level of consciousness that emerges when habitual patterns are broken, necessary to access alternative ways of seeing and even new creative energy. While the pandemic makes us realize how fragile and inattentive (because automatic) to life our habitual actions are, the psychedelic revival is symptomatic of a collective striving to become more attentive to life 'where the habits formed in action find their way up to the sphere of speculation' (16) and for understanding afresh how the human and nonhuman are profoundly connected. Both phenomena, the pandemic and the 'return' of psychedelics, resonate with the philosophy of Deleuze and Guattari. The coronavirus operates rhizomatically, by cross-species and cross-border contamination, spanning the entire globe in a vast network, asking us to rethink the place of the human in relation to all kinds of nonhuman agents (earth forces and elements, invisible viruses, climate change, technology that surpasses human understanding and control such as AI and nanotechnology). At the same time, the physical limitations of the various lockdowns and other global pandemic measures have opened more interior spaces and inner journeys that are typical for psychedelic trips and that take us virtually to different dimensions of the human and nonhuman world. The premise of this chapter is that Deleuze and Guattari offer important conceptual tools to make sense of the renewed interest in psychedelics in the context of today's world, against the background of the pandemic and various other crises that we are facing in the epoch of the Anthropocene. The connections between Deleuze and Guattari and the Anthropocene have been evaluated elsewhere more broadly (Saldanha and Stark 2016). The emphasis in this chapter will be on the ethico-aesthetic dimensions of psychedelics that are meaningful but so-far undervalued in the current discourse surrounding the psychedelic revival. More specifically, Deleuze's Bergsonian-inspired cinema theory will be informative for the arguments put forward.

Psychedelics, entheogenic plants and other substances with altering states capacities have been around for ages: shamanistic ayahuasca practices in the Amazon, psilocybin medicines used by curanderos in Mexico, iboga initiations and other religious rites in African cultures, alchemical traditions across the world, esotericism and witch burning in Europe – these are all practices that carry diverse ancient wisdoms of plants, medicine and mind manifesting insights that have not been invented by the Flower Power movement in the United States and Europe in the 1960s (Eliade 1978; Cotnoir 2006; Alpert et al. 2010; Ramey 2012; Hanegraaff 2013). Yet, when we speak of a psychedelic revival, the historic reference is to the wave in popular use of psychedelics in the West during the mid-twentieth century that (arguably) started with the invention of LSD in 1948 by Albert Hofmann, and spread via the medical circuit and the CIA into the general population and popular culture (Martin and Shain 1985; Langlitz 2013; Pollan 2018; Hartogsohn 2020).

This first popular psychedelic wave is generally associated with rebellious and liberating movements: the 1960s counter-culture, the generation gap and the emergence of youth culture, the context of the Cold War and protests against the Vietnam War, emancipation movements such as Women's Lib and the civil rights movement, pop culture (especially music, poster art and iconic movies such as *Easy Rider*, the acid western and other hippie exploitation movies from the West Coast) as well as with avant-garde and experimental movies of the New York and European underground scene (Braunstein and Williams Doyle, 2002; DeAngelis 2018; Pisters 2022). When the movement grew too strong and became controversial not only because of misuses and scandals around controversial gurus such as Timothy Leary and Charles Manson but also because of its threats to the establishment, president Nixon declared the War on Drugs in 1972. This did not only put an end to the medical experiments and legal research on psychedelics in medical contexts but also slowly but surely pushed the counter-cultural practices to the margins where they nevertheless continued to develop in relative silence (Greer 2020).

The current psychedelic revival is associated with very different practices and develops in a different setting. In order to avoid the political and other disagreements associated with the freedom fights and rebellious youth culture of the 1960s, since the late 1990s, neuroscientists and medical doctors have picked up research into the beneficial effects of psychedelic and empathogenic substances (such as ayahuasca, psylocibin and MDMA) under strict medico-ethical and scientific conditions, with a focus on healing and treatment of (what now, not unproblematically, is considered as) brain disorders such as PTSD and severe depression (Langlitz 2013). The larger contextual milieu in which these researches are taking place has also changed. While pop culture is still very important, we now are surrounded by digital networks, big data surveillance, and a growing consciousness of our planetary precariousness, as well as the continued emancipatory fights in #Black Lives Matter and #Metoo global movements (Yusoff 2018; Papasyrou et al. 2019; Williams and Labate 2020).[1] Research and publications on the psychedelic revival have a strong focus on neuro- and medical sciences, on psychiatry and medical anthropology, and on ethnobotanics or (to a lesser extend) on religious practices.[2] In order to revive the potential of psychedelics, its surrounding discourse has by and large been de-politicized in a sobering approach of 'disenchantment' (Langlitz 2013, 44).

What is not often addressed in contemporary psychedelic research is an in-depth consideration of the philosophical and aesthetic dimensions of the inner journeys and its implied significance that often transgresses medical scientific frameworks. This is where Deleuze and Guattari come in. Their concepts such as rhizomatic thinking and becoming-animal or becoming-plant appear at dispersed places in references to the psychedelic revival; but their ideas have not yet been brought together systematically around this topic[3] (Pokorny 2013; Genn-Bash 2015). Because Deleuze and Guattari have been associated with Mai 68 in France and the rebellious youth culture of the 1960s more broadly, and because there are various explicit references to drugs throughout their work, it is not so surprising to see these connection re-emerge. But how can we make the psychedelic qualities of Deleuze and Guattari explicitly relevant for the current wave of interest in psychedelics? How do drugs change perception, 'even of non-users', as Deleuze and Guattari argue in *A Thousand Plateaus* (1988, 248), and why would this be necessary, especially in (post)pandemic times?

Aesthetics of psychedelics: perception and attention to life

In *The Three Ecologies* (2000) Guattari emphasizes the ethico-political and aesthetic dimensions of his so-called ecosophy. Guattari argues for a tripled ecological approach towards our current condition that takes into account the transversal connections between the environment (or material ecologies), the social and political organization of our interpersonal connections and power structures (social ecologies) and the ideas, desires and states of consciousness (mental ecologies). In his conception of ecology as heterogeneous assemblages he argues that artists 'provide us with the most profound insights into the human condition' (Pindar and Sutton in Guattari 2000, 8). Deleuze, too, has written about art, cinema and literature, and the collaborative work between Deleuze and Guattari is characterized by a prevailing eye on artworks, aesthetics and sense perception. So what insights can we draw from this in understanding the psychedelic renaissance?

If we want to know more about the psychedelic experience as an aesthetic phenomenon, Aldous Huxley's 'trip reports' remain a seminal artistic starting point to recall. In *The Doors of Perception* Huxley describes his mescaline experience with meticulous precision. He recounts how one spring day in 1953 he took a pill at eleven in the morning. An hour and a half later he saw the flowers in the vase on his dining table with new eyes: 'I was seeing what Adam had seen on the morning of his creation – the miracle, moment by moment, of naked existence' (2004, 7). For the first time in his life, Huxley could just see the 'Is-ness' of the flowers, 'shining with their own light', perceiving

> what the rose and iris and carnation signified was nothing more, and nothing less, than what they were – a transience that was yet eternal life, a perpetual perishing that was at the same time pure Being, a bundle of minute, unique particulars in which, by some unspeakable and yet self-evident paradox, was to be seen the divine source of all existence (7).

He describes how he saw the flowers breathing, 'from beauty to heightened beauty, from deeper to even deeper meaning' (7). After that he describes how also the colours of other objects (such as the covers of the books on his shelves) had become so intense that they were intrinsically meaningful: 'they seemed to be on the point of leaving the shelves to thrust themselves more intensely to my attention' (8).

What we see is that the moving inward of the mescaline experience opens the doors to perceiving more attentively the life of nonhuman entities. Also, the experience of place and distance transform in the mescaline experience into a profoundly significant experience of 'intensity of existence' (9). Time equally becomes something altogether different, changing into the experience of a perpetual duration of presence. Compositions become pronounced: Huxley obtains the eye of a 'pure aesthete', beyond the utilitarian spectrum 'whose concern is only with forms and their relationships within the field of vision or picture space' (10). And he adds that his purely aesthetic Cubist-eye view also gave way to a sacramental vision of reality, endowing everything with an inner light. Much of *The Doors of Perception* is a description of art and the ways in which artists are equipped with the power of seeing the expressiveness of the mysteries of pure being in their artwork; 'what the rest of us only see under the influence of mescalin' (18). Van Gogh, Cézanne, Vermeer, Rembrandt, Japanese and Chinese landscape painters, musicians and many more artists are raised by Huxley to describe the profound psychedelic experiences that gave him at the same time a feeling of ethical responsibility and thankfulness towards existence.

From this we can conclude that the aesthetic dimension in a psychedelic journey turns the world into an artwork, and vice versa, it seems that artists are able to capture something of this altered state of reality in their artistic expressions. By emphasizing this direct experience of life in the act of perception, Huxley argues that the world is in profound need of what he calls the 'non-verbal Humanities', 'the arts of being directly aware of the given facts of our existence [which] are almost completely ignored' (48). In *Heaven and Hell* he adds that the otherworldly light and colours that are shared in all visionary experiences have an immediate meaning which is as intense as the colours and light: 'And their meaning consists precisely in this, that they are intensely themselves and, being intensely themselves, are manifestations of essential givenness, the non-human otherness of the universe' (61). What the aesthetics dimension of the psychedelic experience unfolds is perception 'in the midst of things' (Deleuze and Guattari 1987, 282). We encounter here the Bergsonian premise that perception *is* something in itself and not necessarily the perception of something else (a preconceived idea, a recognizable image, a doxa, common sense) (Bergson 1991, 67; Deleuze and Guattari 1994, 149–150). Also, the direct attention to the nonhuman otherness of the universe seems to hold importance that is hard to describe in words, but can be felt and sensed in certain aesthetic experiences.

Ontology of intensity at the limits of perception

Let me move a bit deeper down the rabbit hole to find some more general aesthetic characteristics of the psychedelic experience. Huxley acknowledges that every psychedelic, visionary or mystic experience is unique, but he also insists that they share certain patterns and characteristics (Huxley 2004, 63).[4] In *American Trip* Ido Hartogsohn argues that the highly malleable and singular effects of drugs (that for large parts depend on set and setting)[5] are possible because of several common aesthetic perceptions and sensations that all belong to what he calls an 'ontology of intensity' (Hartogsohn 2020: 12–13). First, rather than a suppressant (like antidepressants) that dampen experience, all psychedelic drugs tend to magnify, amplify, dramatize and intensify the content of one's experience: details become pronounced, larger or smaller, colours more vivid, sounds louder and closer, emotions deeper. The second fundamental aesthetic characteristic of psychedelics is a hyper associative tendency which manifests and allows for instance synaesthetic perception (tasting colour, seeing touch), and other creative connections between usually dispersed objects or dimensions (for instance time travelling to ancestors, seeing the molecules of a plant, or moving inside the interior design of a machine). A third core aspect of psychedelics is the blurring or melting of boundaries, present at the level of perception (such as flowing or dissolving forms in sight and sound). These perceptive characteristics can also transform into a temporary ego-loss and unification with nature, the cosmos or other people (Huxley's heaven); or, in the scarier version, of the total eclipse of the self, paranoia or confrontation with demons or dragons (hell). All these core elements of the intensified ontology of psychedelics manifest in variegated ways in response to different sets and settings, forming multiple feedback loops between the effects of psychedelic substances and society and culture.[6]

From these general patterns of the psychedelic experience, we can draw that a psychedelic aesthetics opens perception via intense colours and light, synaesthetic mingling of the senses, as well as molecularization and liquification of perception. Mathematical abstractions, geometric figures, fractals and multi-perspectives are part of the psychedelic aesthetic pattern (Hartogsohn 2018). This level of aesthetic abstraction is often joined by another level which is more figurative, often in a weird way, full of bizarre figures, surreal objects or distorted bodies, symbolic images and archetypes that have their own dream logic or Alice in Wonderland-like dimensions. The acknowledgement of the sometimes bizarre and weird encounters that the contents of the psychedelic experience entails, is just as significant as its other more abstract aesthetic elements. As Erik Davis argues:

> Mediating weirdness is particularly true when we consider the question of psychedelic entities, which in some sense is one of the phenomenological elements that are the most unassimilable into the Western framework. You might do yoga and experience oneness or absolute peace with the universe, and you can still square that with what is happening to your endocrine system or blood flow or proprioception. That's fine. But if you have a conversation with a toad in a velvet jacket, there is not a lot of room to move with a materialist framework, except toward the basket of psychosis or hallucination (Davis 2018, 124; see Davis 2019).

This second dimension of psychedelic perception brings us to the more symbolic and perhaps even archetypical aspects of the psychedelic (see Powell 2007; Settle and Worley 2016).

Let us now first zoom in on the ontological intensity of the psychedelic journey and turn to Deleuze, who in *Difference and Repetition* discusses intensity as an experience 'at the limits of perception' (1994, 144) at the point where the quality in the sensible turns into its transcendence (what Deleuze calls empirical transcendentalism). Intensity here is understood as 'pure difference in itself', as that which is 'both imperceptible for empirical sensibility which grasps intensity only already covered or mediated by the quality to which it gives rise, and at the same time that which can be perceived only from the point of view of transcendental sensibility which apprehends it immediately in the encounter' (144). Deleuze adds that when this limit sensibility is transmitted to the imagination, this 'phantasteon' is 'both that which can only be imagined and the empirically unimaginable' (ibid.). As Settle and Worley argue, for Deleuze, sense is an event that takes place 'within the fragile environment of aesthetic affects'. This means that in this liminal aesthetic zone 'sense verges closely on becoming non-sense' (Settle and Worley 2016, 8). In all cases, whether in abstract perception or in weird phantasteons of more figurative imagination, all begins with sensibility, with being able to perceive, to pick up intensities which opens doors of perception and allows new thoughts to emerge, precisely because it might be weird or eerie, 'that which lies beyond standard perception [which is] often a sign that we are in the presence of something new' (Fisher 2016, 8, 13). The differential in thought arrives through an encounter with intensity. Psychedelics are mediators of such intensities that are at the core of Deleuze's ontology that, I have to say upfront, not necessarily depends on psychedelics but certainly resonates with its aesthetics. We have to recall here Deleuze's quote from William Burroughs in the *Logic of Sense*: 'Imagine that everything that can be attained by chemical means is accessible by other paths . . . oh psychedelia' (Deleuze 1990, 161). And Deleuze and Guattari's reminder in *A Thousand Plateaus* that it is important to succeed on getting drunk on pure water (Deleuze and Guattari 1988, 286). I will return to the explicit references to the use of drugs further on. But let me first turn to Deleuze's take on perception in cinema.

The nonhuman camera eye

One of the reasons why Deleuze is interested in cinema is precisely because of its 'psychedelic' potentiality to offer a perceptual field of intensities (percepts and affects) that take us beyond strictly human phenomenology. Deleuze's Bergsonian cinema project takes film as a means for exploring aesthetic sensation as nonhuman and unnatural perception. In this way, cinema is not an apparatus that reproduces an illusionary perception of reality but quite differently becomes 'the organ for perfecting the new reality' (Deleuze 1986, 8). As is well known, in *The Movement-Image* Deleuze transfers Bergson's view on perception to construct cinema as 'machine assemblage of matter-images' (85). He discusses how the image and the perception of the image is the same thing; perception is the image. While all movement-images combine perception-images, affection-images and action-images, it is important to note that perception-images are not only part of the matter-image assemblages, but in a way they are also primordial to any perception at all, a sort of zero degree of cinema. All cinematographic perception-images move between two extremes: on the one hand, the subjective image, 'seen by someone who forms part of the set' (71); on the other hand, the objective image, 'when the thing or the set are seen from the viewpoint of someone who remains external to that set' (71). Deleuze argues that cinematographic images actually always have a supple (free indirect) status oscillating between subjective and objective points of view, transformed by a camera consciousness, an inhuman camera eye.

In the perception-image we also encounter the limits of perception at the boundaries of the subjective and objective poles, where the empirical experience of the image encounters its transcendence. On one extreme, Deleuze refers to the liquid perception of the innermost (subjective) pole of perception: the delirium, dream or hallucination. Deleuze mentions among others German expressionism and the French school of water in the cinema of filmmakers such as Jean Renoir, Jean Epstein and Jean Vigo. In their films the rhythm and liquid abstraction of water signify 'the promise or implication of another state of perception, a more than human perception, a perception not tailored to solids .... A more delicate and vaster perception, a molecular perception, peculiar to a cine eye' (80). At the other limit, Deleuze distinguishes the 'gaseous perception' of the outermost (objective) pole of perception, defined by inhuman editing techniques and impossible camera positions, as in Vertov's cine-eye where the camera and montage bring the nonhuman eye in things. What montage does, according to Vertov, is to carry perception into things, to put perception into matter, so that any point whatsoever in space itself perceives all the points on which it acts, or which act on it, however far these actions and reactions extend. This is the definition of objectivity, 'to see without boundaries or distance' (81). In this sense, cinema reached to the genetic element of all possible perception. Perception now becomes gaseous, 'defined by the free movement of each molecule ... attaining pure perception as it is in things or in matter' (84).

Besides Vertov, Deleuze here also refers to the experimental and underground cinema of Stan Brakhage, Michael Snow and Jordan Belson, who all experiment at the limits of perception via a camera-consciousness. Here Deleuze wonders if drugs can have a similar effect of perceptive experimentation brought about by different means:

> To follow Castaneda's programme of initiation: drugs are supposed to stop the world, to release the perceptions of doing ... to make one see the molecular intervals, the holes in sound, in forms, and even in water ... to make lines of speed pass through these holes in the world ... beyond the solid and [even] the liquid: to reach another perception, which is also the genetic element of all perception (85).

We see here that Deleuze endows the camera with nonhuman perception that at its limits of intensity becomes a means to create a psychedelic aesthetic experience with different, artistic and technological means. So there seems to be a profound connection between the camera, artistic perception and drugs that goes beyond the representation of hippies in altered states of consciousness in exploitations films of the 1960s that are often associated with psychedelics in relation to cinema (Pisters 2022). Media and drugs both operate at the level of renewing perception, opening up the habitual patterns and potentially creating new creative energies.

Here Deleuze's Bergsonian theory of perception offers an insight into the psychedelic revival in our current times of crisis and transformation where we (consciously and unconsciously, individually and collectively) are looking for alternative ways of being in the world. Again, this is not new; also in the first psychedelic wave this link between cultural transformation and mind-altering practices was acknowledged. In a famous interview in *Playboy* in 1969 Marshall McLuhan argues that drugs 'are a natural means of smoothing cultural transitions, and also a short cut into the electric vortex' (McLuhan in Norden 1969, 13). McLuhan was talking about the revolutionary changes caused by electric media and the television (which he famously described as a means of turning the world into a global village):

> Drug taking is stimulated by today's pervasive environment of instant information, with its feedback mechanism of the inner trip ... which are the basic needs of people translated by electric extensions of their central nervous systems out of the old rational, sequential value system. The attraction to hallucinogenic drugs is a means of achieving empathy with our penetrating electric environment, an environment that in itself is a drugless inner trip (13; see also Skinnon 2012).

And so we can see that the psychedelic revival also seems to respond to a time of crisis and transition, where the COVID-19 pandemic has equally given a booster to electronic digital media, ranging from zoom meetings to the frantic search for new technologies that undoubtedly will ask many new forms of perception and understanding to make sense of the increasingly techno-mediated (and in many other ways transformed) world to come.

Revealing bodies without organs of cinema

So far I have spoken about aesthetics at the limits of perception, which is where we encounter intensity and the potential for change and renewal, finding another level in psychic life. But what about the body? Again it is interesting to return one more time to

Deleuze's cinema books and consider the place of the body. Deleuze points out how cinema transcends (or can transcend) common phenomenological embodiment. In *The Time-Image* Deleuze spends several pages on the work of Philippe Garrel and demonstrates how Garrel's cinema, which can be considered psychedelic as I will argue below, creates a level of intensity through his cinematographic treatment and constitution of the body (Deleuze 1989, 198–202). Deleuze analyses how, throughout his work, Garrel always returns to a basic set of bodies: that of the man, the woman and the child, as a sort of sacred genesis of the 'holy trinity'. These returning bodies in Garrel's cinema are not of flesh and blood; often filmed in black and white and treated more as figures in a milieu, 'primordial bodies' that are rather aesthetic gestures. More importantly, they are bodies that do not offer a real human presence (Deleuze refers here to the difference between the presence of actual bodies in theatre and of the absence of such present bodies in cinema). The films of Garrel demonstrate, par excellence, the inhuman quality of cinema yet again at the limits of perception, at the limits of what constitutes a body. It is a cinema that 'works with "dancing seeds" and "luminous dust"; it affects the visible with a fundamental disturbance, and the world with a suspension, which contradicts all natural perception' (201).

Perhaps a brief analysis of two of Garrel's early films, *The Revealer* (1968) and *The Inner Scar* (1972) can make the points mentioned here a little more tangible.[7] Both films have a level of abstraction that makes the experience of watching them quite psychedelic in that they break with the habitual ways of seeing. Shot in black and white and without sound, *The Revealer* (quite literally in terms of staging and camera movement) turns around a four-year-old child (Stanislas Robiolle) and its parents (Laurent Terzieff and Bernadette Lafont) who move through the woods and desolate roads and landscapes, sometimes occupying an empty bedroom. Deleuze recalls 'the fine opening' of the film (199) that presents the three figures in chiaroscuro: first the child (on top of a bunkbed) is revealed in the darkness, its face low key lit; then a door opens and the father becomes visible against a bright white background of the adjacent room; and finally the camera moves downward and the mother appears sitting on the floor in front of the father. Throughout the film we see them moving in geometric patterns, creating lines and points in space, traversing the landscape, running through the woods at night, crawling in barb wired grass, walking towards or away from the camera on a dark, empty, wet road. Their bodies are like moving flecks of lumination in the dark. Sometimes they sit down, the child circling around them. In another scene we just see their heads, placed at three points against a white background in the shape of a triangle. There is a sense of dread, of persecution. But also a sense of caring for each other, and of loss. The child remains enigmatic. In a haunting scene we see the child in the back of a driving truck or a car, crop dusting some kind of gas from a spray can out the window. In the background in blurred focus, along the driving car, the parents run along, reaching out to the unattainable child. The film ends with the child alone by the sea.

The Revealer is filmed at the limits of perception: in silence, in under and overexposed black-and-white film stock, with only three characters that perform gestures and poses and trace lines or figures rather than act in any kind of realistic way. And yet, precisely because of all these limited conditions, the film becomes some kind of hallucinatory experience in itself. It penetrates the mind of the spectator who becomes aware of their own thoughts, their own bodies (and bodily sounds) and aware of the enfolded layers of the different 'Bodies without Organs' that the film presents: besides the trinity of the child, the man and the woman, there is the trinity of the filmmaker, the characters and the camera that is revealed. In a long sequence where the man, the woman and the child crawl and sneak through the high grass (their gestures make them enter into a becoming-animal), the camera sometimes follows them directly, sometimes waits for the characters to move forward to catch up with them a moment later. And at one point the child waves at the filmmaker behind the camera, inviting him to follow them through the grass. We see here perception transformed through camera consciousness. 'Revealer', *le révélateur* of the French title, refers to the procedure of developing film negatives, and as such the child is also the revealing element of the film that makes visible the sometimes incomprehensible affects and percepts that are presented.[8] The film is shot in post-war Munich, where the spirit of the persecutions still lingered in the woods, and the disillusions of the post-Mai 68 revolutions are tangible in the (often intoxicated and heroine infused) bodies of the crew and cast, even if in the film itself there are no direct references to drugs. Nevertheless, one senses all these levels insisting and persisting onto the limited images on screen.

The Inner Scar (*La cicatrice intérieure*, 1972) is one of the few colour films of Garrel. Again we have the primordial set of bodies here of a woman (Nico), a man (Philippe Garrel, who after the first scenes is replaced by Pierre Clementi) and a child (Christian Päffgen, Nico's real-life son). The film is shot in the hot deserts of New Mexico and Egypt and on the icy black rocks of Iceland. Again most of the movements of the bodies form geometric points, lines and especially circles. At the beginning of the film the woman is wailing, enfolded in the desert rocks, almost blending into the geology of the earth, when the man (Garrel) approaches from far, and takes her away. She sinks down onto the sandy desert floor, and he walks away. The camera keeps on following him in a travelling shot to the left, until we realize he has returned to the point where he left the woman and thus made a circle. As such, bodies are points tracing lines and figures, often accompanied by Nico's singing voice.[9] While the abstract figures and patterns gain the ontological intensity that is part of a psychedelic aesthetic, *The Inner Scar* also addresses a more weird symbolism. The elements carry material and symbolic value: earthly grounding of the sand and the rocks, burning circles of fire, water in the form of ice and the sea, and air as white skies and (lack of) breathing space; there are also horses and a small boat that carries Clementi, naked, holding a sword. On this level the images are surreal, symbolic and mystical. They are to be taken as a feverish dream, again indicating how drugs operate at the level of artistic creation of new perception.

In a way we could say that cinema, in any case certain types of cinema that are not representational, produces quite literally Bodies without Organs, in that they become purely gestural, and produces new ways of organizing or composing the body. Garrel's films produce a choreography of bodies that turn around the child as a problematic point, 'an empty turning point, unattainable limit, or irrational cut', as Deleuze observes (199). Moreover, the films of Garrel are hallucinatory and psychedelic, not only because actors, characters and filmmakers were often under the influence of substances (ranging from heroin to opium and weed) but precisely because the camera captures unhabitual forms of perception, returning its observations back to the spectators. It is a cinema that returns to abstract geometry such as lines and circles, but also alterations of over- and underexposure, hot and cold ('heat of the fire or a light in the night, the cold of the white drug' [200]) that compose the strange cinematographic bodies that penetrate our perception, provoking altered states of consciousness in a similar way to how substances can.

Knights of narcotics and black holes of dependency

Because of the experimentations with drugs (both off-screen and sometimes shown on-screen, like the heroin addiction of the woman in *The Secret Son* (1970) or the opium smoking of the friends in *Regular Lovers* (2005)), Garrel could also be called a 'knight of narcotics' that Deleuze and Guattari mention in *A Thousand Plateaus* (1988):

> These knights claim that drugs, under necessary conditions of caution and experimentation, are inseparable from the deployment of a plane ... [where] the imperceptible itself becomes necessarily perceived at the same time as perception becomes necessarily molecular [and] invests desire directly: arrive at holes, micro-intervals between matters, colours and sounds engulfing lines of flight, world lines .... Change perception (282).

So drugs, for Deleuze and Guattari, can be understood at the level of the direct investment in perception, opening new doors of perception indeed. They speak of a 'pharmacoanalysis' that immediately addresses an immanent 'perception-consciousness system' where experimentation replaces interpretation (of the Unconscious of psychoanalysis): 'Drugs give the unconscious an immanence that psychoanalysis has constantly botched' (284).

However, Deleuze and Guattari do not simply promote the use of drugs as such because, they warn, there is a danger of dependence on 'the hit, the dose, the dealer' (284). and more importantly of the possibility of the black hole of self-destruction ('each addict a hole') where the making of a rich body without organs full of intensities, gives way to an emptied or 'vitrified body that turns into a line of death' (285). Drugs are too unwieldy, Deleuze and Guattari argue, to guarantee a vital life-assemblage. They do not reject psychedelia and other substances, but they maintain that the issue with drugs is to reach the point where 'to get high or not to get high' is no longer the question, but rather 'whether drugs have sufficiently changed the general conditions of perception so that nonusers can succeed passing through the holes in the world' (286). Film can be one of the possible ways of investing perception directly. But here again, we also have to acknowledge that film (and other media forms) may pose their own forms of addiction (McKenna 1992; Enns 2006; MacDougall 2012; Alter 2017). One of the most compelling films in which drug addiction, *and* addiction to the film camera, directly invests the field of perception via the nonhuman eye, is the Spanish cult classic *The Rapture* (*Arrebato*, Ivan Zulueta, 1980). It is worthwhile recalling this film before returning to the contemporary context of the psychedelic revival.

The Rapture's main character is a Madrilene horror film director José Sirgado (Eusebio Poncela) who receives a package with a super8 film and audiocassette from a cousin of his ex-girlfriend Pedro (Will More). José has a tumultuous relationship with his girlfriend Ana Turner (Cecilia Roth), but the film does not care about these plot details. Rather it is a deep and disturbing aesthetic and ontological investigation of the power of the camera. References to the horror genre constitute one level to raise this power of the camera: the camera is the vampire, and once 'bitten' there is no way of stopping, to the point of rapture (whether this is a mystical experience or death). However, the film digs deeper into what the camera itself can reveal of so many hidden and unperceivable dimensions of reality itself. Explicitly acknowledged are reflections on places never visited before, speeds, rhythms, dimensions never perceived with the human eye; but now, with the help of the camera, are felt and experienced. One can notice throughout the film how this power of the camera to change and transform perception is influenced by and resonates with the psychedelic experiences at the time. But we also enter the much darker, disturbing sides of this rapturing power of cinema. The characters (like the actors at the time) use heroin and are equally addicted to the image in a non-metaphoric way: scoring a film, withdrawal symptoms while waiting for the next development of a reel; the relations between drugs and cinema are direct. Self-referentiality to cinema equipment (cameras, sound recorders, projectors, film strips, editing equipment, film posters) are everywhere in Zulueta's film.

Most striking is the desire to be totally absorbed by the camera: 'I wanted a relationship exclusively produced through film, shooting, projection,' Pedro confesses on an audiotape. Moreover, the camera seems to develop a life of its own. Pedro discovers that it has started filming him while he is asleep. When he has the film developed, he notices that his portrait image is slowly but surely being absorbed by red frames; to the point where he disappears completely, not only on the film but also in reality. A dissolution of identity, raptured by the camera. *The Rapture* is a total cinephile love story about the frenzy of the visible empowered by the camera that is destructive, inviting self-effacement and ego-loss. So in its essence, this weird and eerie but fascinating film is about the ontology of the camera eye and its aesthetics of transforming perception that completely interpenetrates reality. Like drugs, it invests desire directly into the limits of perception, rendering it molecular, opening up to the imperceptible.

The esoteric circle: nonhuman ethics and restoring a belief in the world

And thus, taking into account the dangers of any limited experience, the immanent power of cinema and psychedelics alike is valued by Deleuze and Guattari as an essential quality for the emergence and creation of the new, which always involves a hermetic mystery. As Joshua Ramey explains, in valuing artists in this esoteric way, 'at work here is a deeply ethical program, in the Spinozistic sense of ethics as expansion of what a body can do' (Ramey 2012, 149). Artistic and psychedelic experiments can bring about change, or restore a belief in the world. Huxley was rather prosaic when he addressed the transformative powers of the psychedelic experience:

> But the man [sic] who comes back through the Door in the Wall will never be quite the same as the man who went out. He will be wiser but less cocksure, happier but less self-satisfied, humbler in acknowledging his ignorance yet better equipped to understand the relationship of words to things, of systematic reasoning to the unfathomed Mystery which it tries, forever vainly, to comprehend (Huxley 2004, 50).

In Garrel's work we can see that the circles his characters draw are often 'esoteric circles' (one of the chapters in *The Secret Son* is explicitly called 'The Ophidian Circle' that contains a secret door to hidden wisdom at the limits of experience), which Deleuze raises as the hermetic symbolism for eternal return of the new (1994, 91). In *The Time-Image* he argues that Garrel's cinema is a 'cinema of constitution' that can 'restore our belief in the world' (Deleuze 1989, 201), which ultimately is the only ethical mission of cinema and art more generally, according to Deleuze and Guattari.

So, to conclude, I want to return to the psychedelic revival, and the question of what Deleuze and Guattari have to offer in understanding the psychedelic revival. As indicated at the beginning, the renewed interest in psychedelics is no longer predominantly about freedom and rebellion but rather about healing and reconnecting to forms of life that we have by and large been inattentive to. It is not only to find new treatment for depression and other wounds of our individual brains and collective mental life, but also more generally, as Ronan Hallowell point out, about finding remedies for a wounded world (Hallowell 2012, 251; Badiner 2017). In *What Is Philosophy?* Deleuze and Guattari attribute aesthetics with medicinal qualities, revealing genetic and regenerative elements: 'elements that, as virtual, are not directly experienced in sensation, yet constitute the being of the sensible in the precise sense that imperceptible vibrations constitute the being of every colour' (Ramey 2012, 152). Art therefore points to the 'anorganic life within life' and aesthetics (affects, percepts) point to these 'nonhuman dimensions and becomings of man' (Deleuze and Guattari 1994, 169).

What Deleuze and Guattari can offer is a philosophical understanding of the psychedelic experience as aesthetic experience at the limits of perception that points to a radical ethics. Andrew Lapworth designates this ethics as a 'responsibility before the world' that is ontogenetic in that it raises explicitly the question of new ways of seeing and thinking that include the nonhuman (2021). The ethical dimension of the aesthetics of the psychedelic experience is that it goes beyond the human condition, offering what Vivieros de Castro has called perspectivism (2014). As Lapworth points out, perspectivism is different from relativism, as the latter always remains in relation to a (human) centred point of view, while perspectivism is a-central and actually immanent to (human and nonhuman) entities and (molecular, imperceptible) forces that are part of the world (2021, 396). While Deleuze saw the radical ethics of such a-centred perception embodied in *The Time-Image* and the return to the experimental films of Garrel and Zulueta that I have recalled in this chapter, contemporary cinema may offer its own experiments. Here I could mention for instance another revival, the renewed interest in the horror genre and a poetics of horror that is significantly renewed in women directors from diverse ethnic and cultural backgrounds. Mati Diop's *Atlantics*

(2019) and Julia Ducournau's *Titane* (2021) would be cases in point to look at a renewed horror aesthetics and radical ethics of the nonhuman, be it the deceased or cars (Pisters 2020). But this would take another essay. For now, I wanted to return to the writings and set and setting in which Deleuze and Guattari developed their work and demonstrate how in the context of a (post)pandemic world, where we are living with these invisible nonhuman forces, the wisdom of plants and chemical substances operate directly on the senses, taking them to the limits of perception where we may find ways to restore our belief in the world, perhaps the most radical meaning of the aesthetics of the psychedelic experience.

Notes

1 In spite of the increasing acknowledgements of the need for a decolonizing perspective on the psychedelic revival, and the revaluing of indigenous knowledge and wisdom, the psychedelic revival by and large is still is a 'white western' research field. While elsewhere I address this issue more explicitly (Pisters 2022), here I am not addressing these political dimensions explicitly (while being fully aware that aesthetics is not independent of issues of power, nor is it a neutral philosophical concept).

2 See for instance https://open-foundation.org/ and https://chacruna.net/ for an overview of current (domains of) publications on psychedelics.

3 A special issue on Deleuze and Guattari and the Psychedelic Renaissance of *Deleuze and Guattari Studies* is in preparation at the moment of this writing and will appear in 2022.

4 Huxley (2023) refers among others to *The Tibetan Book of the Dead*. See also Timothy Leary's classic descriptions of the psychedelic experience based on this ancient Tibetan text (Leary, Metzner and Alpert 2008).

5 After Timothy Leary in 1961 introduced the concepts of *set* and *setting* in psychedelic experiments, they have become an integral part of psychedelic practices and discourse. Set, or mind set, refers to personality, expectation and intention of the person taking a psychedelic substance. Setting indicates the social, physical and cultural environment in which the experience takes place (Leary et al., 2008).

6 In this way, Hartogsohn demonstrates that the notorious bad trip became more prominent as an experience 'after the media started to report more on this phenomena and societal and political consensus moved towards the war on drugs' (2020, 206).

7 I would like to thank Jeffrey Babcock for showing this film in his Underground Cinema Program in Amsterdam under covid conditions in the winter of 2021.

8 In *The Secret Son* (*L'enfant secret*, 1979) the child is equally connected to the act of filming. The child (Xuan Lindenmeyer) is the child of the woman (Anne Wiazemsky), who has a love affair with the man (Henri de Maublanc) who is a filmmaker (his 'secret child' is the film he makes). This film is more narrative in that it presents Garrel's decade-long engagement with Velvet Underground Singer Nico (who had an unacknowledged son with Alain Delon). The man in the film is hospitalized and treated with electroshock therapy against depression; the woman acknowledges her heroin addiction at the end of the film.

9 The songs (written and performed by Nico) are 'Abschied', 'Janitor of Lunacy', 'My Only Child', 'All That Is My Own' and 'König'.

References

Alpert, Richard (Ram Dass), Ralph Metzer and Gary Bravo (2010), *Birth of a Psychedelic Culture: Conversations about Leary, The Harvard Experiments, Millbrooks and the Sixties*. Synergetic Press.

Alter, Adam (2017), *Irresistible: The Rise of Addictive Technology and the Business of Keeping Us Hooked*. Penguin Press.

Badiner, Allan (2017), 'Psychedelics in the Anthropocene', in Ben Sessa et al., eds. *Breaking Convention: Psychedelic Pharmacology for the 21st Century*. Strange Attractor Press, 13–20.

Bergson, Henri (1991), *Matter and Memory*. Trans. N. M. Paul and W. S. Palmer. Zone Books.

Braunstein, Peter and Michael Williams Doyle, eds. (2002), *Imagine Nation: The American Counterculture of the 1960s and 1970s*. Psychology Press.

Cotnoir, Brian (2006), *The Weiser Concise Guide to Alchemy*. Weiser Books.

Davis, Erik (2018), 'How to Think Weird Beings' in David Luke and Rory Spowers, eds. *DMT Dialogues: Encounter with the Spirit Molecule*. Park Street Press, 118–153.

Davis, Erik (2019), *High Weirdness: Drugs, Esoterica, and Visionary Experience in the Seventies*. Strange Attractor Press.

DeAngelis, Michael (2018), *Rx Hollywood: Cinema and Therapy in the 1960*. State University of New York.

Deleuze, Gilles (1986), *Cinema 1: The Movement-Image*. Trans. Hugh Tomlinson and Barbara Habberjam. The Athlone Press.

Deleuze, Gilles (1989), *Cinema 2: The Time-Image*. Trans. Hugh Tomlinson and Robert Galeta. The Athlone Press.

Deleuze, Gilles (1990), *The Logic of Sense*. Trans. Mark Lester with Charels Stivale. Columbia University Press.

Deleuze, Gilles (1994), *Difference and Repetition*. Trans. Paul Patton. The Athlone Press.

Deleuze, Gilles and Félix Guattari (1987), *A Thousand Plateaus: Capitalism and Schizophrenia*. Trans. Brian Massumi. The Athlone Press.

Deleuze, Gilles and Félix Guattari (1994), *What Is Philosophy?* Trans. Graham Burchell and Hugh Tomlinson. The Athlone Press.

Eliade, Mircea (1978), *The Forge and the Crucible: The Origins and Structures of Alchemy*. 2nd Edition. Trans. Stephen Corrin. The University of Chicago Press.

Enns, Anthony (2006), 'Media, Drugs and Schizophrenia in the Works of Philip K. Dick', *Science Fiction Studies*, vol. 33, no. 1, 68–88.

Fisher, Mark (2016), *The Weird and the Eerie*. Repeater Books.

Genn-Bash, Oli (2015), 'Deleuze and Psychedelic Thought as Resistance', Dave King et al., eds. *Neurotransmissions: Essays on Psychedelics from Breaking Conventions*. Strange Attractor Press.

Greer, Christian (2020), *Angel-Headed Hipsters: Psychedelic Militancy in Nineteen-Eighties North America*. PhD Thesis, University of Amsterdam.

Guattari, Félix (2008), *The Three Ecologies*. Trans. Ian Pindar and Paul Sutton. Continuum.

Hallowell, Ronan (2012), 'Media Ecological Psychopharmacosophy: An Ecology of the Mind for Today', Robert C. MacDougall, ed. *Drugs and Media: New Perspectives on Communication, Consumption, and Consciousness*. Continuum, 237–265.

Hanegraaff, Wouter (2013), *Western Esotericism*. Bloomsbury.

Hartogsohn, Ido (2018), 'Towards a Science of Psychedelic Aesthetics', Psychedelic Press Blog, 20 December.

Hartogsohn, Ido (2020), *American Trip. Set, Setting, and the Psychedelic Experience in the Twentieth Century*. The MIT Press.
Huxley, Aldous (2004), *The Doors of Perception & Heaven and Hell*. Vintage Classics.
Jodorowsky, Alexander (2010), *Psychomagic: The Transformative Power of Shamanic Psychotherapy*. Inner Traditions Bear and Company.
Langlitz, Nicolas (2013), *Neuropsychedelia: The Revival of Hallucinogen Research since the Decade of the Brain*. University of California Press.
Lapworth, Andrew (2021), 'Responsibility before the World: Cinema, Perspectivism and a Nonhuman Ethics of Individuation', *Deleuze and Guattari Studies*, vol. 15, no. 3, 386–410.
Leary, Timothy, Ralph Metzner and Richard Alpert (2008), *The Psychedelic Experience: A Manual Based on the Tibetan Book of the Dead*. Penguin Classics.
Lee, Martin and Bruce Shain (1985), *Acid Dreams: The Compete Social History of LSD, The CIA, The Sixties, and Beyond*. Grove Press.
MacDougall, Robert, ed. (2012) *Drugs and Media: New Perspectives on Communication, Consumption, and Consciousness*. Continuum, 237–265.
McKenna, Terrence (1992), *Food of the Gods*, Rider.
Norden, Eric (1969), 'The Playboy Interview: A Candid Conversation with the High Priest of Popcult and Metaphysics of Media', *Playboy*, March 1969. Online: The Playboy Interview: Marshall McLuhan (hannemyr.com). Accessed 7 January 2022.
Papasyrou, Maria, Chiara Baldini and David Luke, eds. (2019), *Psychedelic Mysteries of the Feminine*. Park Street Press.
Pisters, Patricia (2020), *New Blood in Contemporary Cinema: Women Directors and the Poetics of Horror*. Edinburgh University Press.
Pisters, Patricia (2022), 'Set and Setting of the Brain on Hallucinogen. Psychedelic Revival in the Acid Western'. Flora Lysen and Stephan Besser, eds. *Worlding the Brain*, Brill.
Pokorny, Vit (2013), 'Biophenomenology of Altered States'. Cameron Adams et al. eds. *Breaking Convention: Essays on Psychedelic Consciousness*. Strange Attractor Press, 197–208.
Pollan, Michael (2018), *How to Change Your Mind: The New Science of Psychedelics*. Allen Lane/Penguin.
Powell, Anna (2007), *Deleuze, Altered States and Film*. Edinburgh University Press.
Ramey, Joshua (2012), *The Hermetic Deleuze: Philosophy and the Spiritual Ordeal*. Duke University Press.
Richards, William (2016), *Sacred Knowledge: Psychedelics and Religious Experiences*. Columbia University Press.
Saldanha, Arun and Hannah Stark, eds. (2016) *Deleuze and Guattari in the Anthropocene*. *Deleuze Studies*, vol. 10. no. 4.
Settle, Zachary and Taylor Worley, eds. (2016), *Dreams, Dread and Doubt. Film and Spirituality*. Cascade Books.
Skinnon, John (2012), 'Psychoactive Media'. Robert Macdougall, ed. *Drugs & Media: New Perspectives on Communication, Consumption, and Consciousness*. Continuum, 66–291.
Viveiros de Castro, Eduardo (2014), *Cannibal Metaphysics*. Trans. Peter Skafish, Universal Publishing.
Williams, Monica and Beatriz Labate, eds. (2020), 'Diversity, Equity, and Access in Psychedelic Medicine', *Journal of Psychedelic Studies*, vol. 4, no. 1.
Yusoff, Kathryn (2018), *A Billion Black Anthropocenes of None*. University of Minnesota Press.

7

Deleuze and Guattari: The Pandemic, the Trump Presidency and the Schizo-Analytic Essay Machine

Damian Ward Hey

The essay machine

My project, here, is to build what Deleuze and Guattari (hereafter referred to as the plural common noun DG) might call a 'schizo-analytic essay machine' that produces a rhizomal critique of several elements of our current ideo-political-socio-economic-etcetera-etcetera-etcetera (ad infinitum) environment. This 'rhizomal critique' is actually itself a producer of desiring in that it seeks further synthesis within the realms of academe or, barring these, any context with which it can find a connection. This blank sheet of paper is a Body without Organs (henceforth BwO) onto which I gradually, asymptotically, place machines of production – desiring machines – that will, by virtue and necessity of that placement in the production of an essay machine, produce an argument machine, which will then form a synthesis – whether connective, conjunctive or disjunctive – with the critical machine that reads it, and so on.

Machines, synthesis and desiring

DG see everything as machines: the mouth machine, the breast machine, the nipple machine, etc. Machines link to other machines in a process called *synthesis*, which may result in three different interrelationships – connective, conjunctive and disjunctive. The purpose of the machine is to produce desiring, which DG define as 'the set of *passive syntheses* that engineer partial objects, flows, and bodies, and that function as units of production' (*The Desiring Machines*, 492). The connective synthesis creates a flow of desiring in which there is undifferentiated unity between production process and product. Although DG categorize this synthesis as pre-capitalist, it can also refer to cooperative, non-hierarchical social models such as hunter-gatherers – models in which there is little if any division of labour. The disjunctive synthesis, by contrast, implements disunity – division of labour, hierarchy, etc. – and is found with industrialism. Finally, the conjunctive synthesis exists in the age of the individual and in which the individual subject can dissolve as quickly as it appears, primarily depending upon that individual subject's ability to produce capital. Thus, this is the synthesis associated with capitalism.

These machines, however, can only be organized to enable synthesis, and therefore desiring, if they attach to a body without organs. Imagine a space, empty of anything that would define it. Add grass and dirt, and the space becomes a field. Add people (who become footballers), a ball (that becomes a football), and a couple of nets while implementing the rules of football, and the empty space of potentiality – the Body without Organs – conforms to the desiring machines (person, ball, goals, rules, etc.) that attach to it. While the game is taking place, the BwO becomes a playing field. When the game, and its artifacts are taken away, the field becomes, once again, a BwO. Add to this that each machine is always 1) built of the synthesis between and among other machines, and 2) that there is infinite potential for any machine itself to be taken apart and made into other machines with other properties, other contexts of desiring production.

Within this approach is a connective synthesis of two desiring machines – books, in this case: *Anti-Oedipus* and *A Thousand Plateaus*. On the subject of books, Deleuze and Guattari suggest that:

> There is no difference between what a book talks about and how it is made. Therefore a book also has no object. As an assemblage, a book has only itself, in connection with other assemblages and in relation to other bodies without organs. We will never ask what a book means, as signified or signifier; we will not look for anything to understand in it. We will ask what it functions with, in connection with what other things it does or does not transmit intensities, in which other multiplicities than its own are inserted and metamorphosed, and with what bodies without organs it makes its own converge.

They are speaking in materialist terms and with a material awareness of the world and of ideology. They are, also, being quite playful – in the Barthesian textual sense of play, tension and desire – of the not quite translatable French word *jouissance* – in their evocation of Marx. They tease the reader with the fluid interiority and exteriority of the book as the result of machines that produce not only a book but a condition of desiring. 'How [a book] is made', for Deleuze and Guattari, means not only the assembling and joining together of the binding materials and the paper and the ink, but also the process of coming up with the proper arrangement of letters, punctuation marks, numbers and spaces. And these are the result, the product, made by the analytical machine of the author, combined with a multiplicity of other machines – not the least of which is the pen and its connection with language, the hand of the author, etc. A book, thus constituted, enters into the field or fields of desiring, be those fields critical desiring, linguistic desiring, institutional desiring, and so forth.

> A book exists only through the outside and on the outside. A book itself is a little machine; what is the relation (also measurable) of this literary machine to a war machine, love machine, revolutionary machine, etc.-and an abstract machine that sweeps them along? (Deleuze and Guattari, 'Rhizome', 4).

Deleuze and Guattari call schizo-analytic (as opposed to psycho-analytic or schizophrenic, both terms having been co-opted by the Oedipal) the process of desiring machines achieving desiring with other desiring machines. The desiring machine may be attached to a will, at some point – itself another desiring machine – but the product of that will is not separate from the desiring machine, itself. What they produce is the 'real'.

> If desire produces, its product is real. If desire is productive, it can be productive only in the real world and can produce only reality. Desire is the set of *passive syntheses* that engineer partial objects, flows, and bodies, and that function as units of production. The real is the end product, the result of the passive syntheses of desire as autoproduction of the unconscious. Desire does not lack anything; it does not lack its object. It is, rather, the *subject* that is missing in desire, or desire that lacks a fixed subject; there is no fixed subject unless there is repression. Desire and its object are one and the same thing: the machine, as a machine of a machine. Desire is a machine, and the object of desire is another machine connected to it. Hence the product is something removed or deducted from the process of producing: between the act of producing and the product, something becomes detached, thus giving the vagabond, nomad subject a residuum (Deleuze and Guattari, *The Desiring Machines*, 492).

Yet it should be pointed out, quickly, that if the product (desiring) is removed from the process of producing (producing that desiring), and if it therefore outside – 'detached' – from the desiring machine, that product then has the potential to *become* desiring – that which is an unfixed object. In this way, the cycle of production of desire and the product of desiring is perpetuated. Paradoxically, desiring is ever outside of the desire to produce desiring.

Whether the desire of this essay machine in synthesis with the critical (or analytical) machine is achieved, as well as which form of synthesis is realized, is always an incomplete determination – and one that is, ultimately, irrelevant to itself as a desiring machine. Unlike Oedipal structures that would see in desire a lack – in this case an ultimate conclusive response that signals the exclusion of other systems of coding and analysis, and actively goes about the repression of desiring machines outside of its own framework – this essay machine is schizo-analytical, meaning that it is chiefly concerned with the continuation of the process of producing desiring, and, as Marx would put it, with reproducing the means of production of that desire to produce desiring – that critical desire, that academic or philosophical desire – in this case, ever incompletely labelled as 'The Field of Deleuze and Guattari Studies'. For no field can be said to be complete that is still 'alive', which is to say, still producing ideology and inquiry through the synthesis of desiring machines. Again, however, incompleteness in the current context does not signify lack, but rather further realizable potential for synthesis and desirability.

And yet a contradiction must take place for this desiring machine to function with other machines. Deleuze and Guattari point out that repression in the form of foreclosure is necessary for any sort of synthesis to take place (*Anti-Oedipus*, 160).

However, even as this repression is oriented toward a diversity of potential contexts, each desiring machine must limit its machine partner in synthesis, this repression, this 'limitation', takes place upon a body without organs whose potential is, by definition unlimited – or, better, *non*-limited. Therefore, though each desiring machine may potentially choose from among an infinity of other machines, its placement upon the body without organs requires a choice, a limitation, (a repression devoid of repression) in order to become inscribed upon that body without organs in a meaningful way – and in this example, 'meaning' refers to the ability to produce either desire or desiring.

The universal history of BwO and desiring machines

Deleuze and Guattari recognize the presence of the Body without Organs and the production of desiring by desiring machines, first and foremost, as universal history. Both the Body without Organs and desiring machines are ever-present and unchanging in their function, regardless of way nature, technology or society manifest them. Deleuze and Guattari recognize The Body of the Earth as the first producer of everything – all material before its use-value is coded by humans. In what previous generations would have called an act of heresy, they displace human autonomy – that which Genesis refers to as mankind's 'stewardship' over the earth and its creatures – and relegate humankind, individual humans, to being part of a social machine. As such, humans are not removed from nature and placed in a position of dominion, centrality, and stewardship over the earth, but are instead re-understood as machines produced by the array of machines that the earth, itself a machine, produces.

Humans, both individual and collective, are therefore desiring machines that produce and sustain the realm of technology. I use the word 'realm' in the broad sense of the space of everything related to production and product – e.g. the technological realm, the social realm, the political realm, etc. I stop short of calling a realm a BwO because by virtue of being labelled the realm has already lost the non-status of a BwO that it had once had. The social realm is also that which produces ideology and economic systems through which to implement that ideology. (And here, DG have referred to the social realm as the result of a conforming 'socius' which up until being connected to desiring machines had itself been a BwO.)

The importance of Marxist materialism to the philosophical production of Deleuze and Guattari cannot be overestimated, other than to ascribe to it a tyrannical and totalizing purview. Desire and desirability result from physical commodities interacting and synthesizing. That which exists in the world of Deleuze and Guattari exists as a compound structure made of other machines – or, put another way, as a machine made of other machines. And, as this structure is built of an essentially non-directed schizo process, the world that is produced – the landscape and array of potential theories and practices produced – is not unified. As a result, in order to best serve the conditioning of desiring, the desiring machines follow a schizo process that takes account of every stimulus, every flow, every pattern of flow (if only to reject them) – and in this way, the schizo, themselves a machine, has greater recourse to variety and disunity, than to the monolith and restriction placed upon the world by a tyrannical

Oedipal discourse. Note well, however, that although DG do not ascribe to Oedipal psychoanalysis, nor to any other totalizing discourse in full – including Marxism – neither do they disavow its validity nor attempt to dismantle its components. They simply call into question its universal application and encourage everyone to pick and choose among a variety of other discourses.

Schizo-analytic instead of psycho-analytic

This last statement, put another way, is that Deleuze and Guattari with humanity to get up from the psycho-analytic couch and to re-vitalize themselves by taking a walk outside as a schizo, able to take in the whole multi-discursive world in which the world immerses them, and to be able to free in their choice rather than bound by Oedipus. The central schizo-analytic project of *Anti-Oedipus* and of DG's work, in general throughout *Anti-Oedipus* and *A Thousand Plateaus* is to dismantle totalizing discourses and the tyranny they bring about.

Anti-Oedipus presents the Oedipal as the most urgent of the totalizing discourses to eschew and to dismantle through the schizo-analytical project because of its predominance within our world – a predominance that they recognize as an international industry of its own self-promotion and continuance rather than an effective therapeutic aid to the individual or collective human psyche.

> Oedipus is indeed the limit, but the displaced limit that now passes into the interior of the socius. Oedipus is the baited image with which desire allows itself to be caught (*That*'s what you wanted! The decoded flows were incest!) … Territorial representation comprises these three instances: the *repressed representative*, the *repressing representation*, and the *displaced represented* (*Anti-Oedipus*, 166).

The face of Oedipus, Deleuze and Guattari assert, has been placed upon every aspect (every *practical* aspect) of power relationship in our socius – that BwO moulded into place for the organization of the desiring machines of human affairs.

In *Anti-Oedipus*, the schizo-analytic rejection all of the codes, laws, restrictions, etc. that Oedipus has forced upon the socius, along with the construction of the schizo-analytic in opposition to the psychoanalytic, is wholly codified by Marxist materialism and posits the physical world as reality (composed of body without organs and non-coded freely-associating desiring production). By embracing a materialist awareness rather than, say an Hegelian one, DG emphasize the practical over the theoretical. Machines of synthesis – essentially of materialist dialectic – construct everything. By overcoming those discourses that would over-ride them, human freedom of choice and will is facilitated. The term 'schizo' is given a positive, open, explorational connotation rather than the pathological one generally ascribed to it by medicine and psychology. Yet, reflective of this schizo orientation, DG resist formulating their Marxist sensibilities as themselves a totalizing discourse. (It would, therefore, be acceptable – although, according to Deleuze and Guattari counterproductive – for the schizo to approach the world as though it were *not* entirely the product of the syntheses of materialist dialectic desiring machines.)

The caveat in producing an essay machine is to be aware that through the very act of production, a codifying system is placed over the text for the purpose of adding itself to (and potentially finding synthesis with) the network of other essay machines on Deleuze and Guattari that are present not only in the current volume but also, by potential schizo-association, with other essays and analytical machines in the Deleuze and Guattari industry (to extend the machine analogy to its vulgar extreme). Deleuze and Guattari's text is, itself, unable to escape becoming a potential machine for theoretical blindness and exclusion so far as the theorist, whether schizo or Oedipal, Marxist or Hegelian, uses and is guided by the language machine, the ordering machine, the analytical machine, the textual machine, etc. Where there is choice, there is also overdeterminism and exclusion. Where there is codification, there is also the bias of discernment.

This essay machine now adds to the previous discussion of desiring machines to suggest that the rhizomal and the arborescent, as presented in 'Rhizome', the introductory essay to *Mille Plateaux* [A Thousand Plateaus] are both formed by the developing, evolving networks of synthesized and synthesizing desiring machines. Thus, there is a bridge created from one Deleuzean paradigm of desiring flow to another. And yet the synapse between the two paradigms is not prohibitively broad. The two are brought together for the practical purpose of understanding the desiring flow – the associative, multi-potential and overdetermined relationship among the discourses of power, politics, and protest evident in the contemporary United States. Ultimately, as with the construction of any desiring machine, this desiring machine can only be incomplete. It can only produce desiring for further synthesis, further understanding, further essay machines to pick up with the production of intellectual desiring where this machine leaves off. (Isn't this the true, open-ended purpose of the bibliography – not only to site the source of information, but also to provide an intertextual point of further departure?)

Rhizomality, arborescence, the Body without Organs and the postmodern president

The well-known trope of arborescent and rhizomal structures of relational flow is useful in understanding of the associative, multi-potential and overdetermined relationship among the discourses of power, politics and protest evident in the United States under former president Donald Trump. The approach, though cursory within in the current space, is guided by the idea that COVID-19 spreads rhizomally yet can be traced arborescently. The presence of rhizomality and arborescence requires a space of cultivation in order to be made manifest and to grow. This space is the Body without Organs. In an attempt to give material expression to an essentially non-material presence, the essay machine recognizes as a Body without Organs that empty, non-defined space of the White House and presidential responsibilities vacated by President Trump after losing the election in the middle of a viral pandemic.

The Deleuzean spread of COVID-19 became politicized by a Trumpian recalcitrance already nascent in the partisan consciousness of the United States before the 2016 presidential election. This recalcitrance was exacerbated under Trump and evolved into partisan tribalism during the four years of his presidency between 2016 and 2020.

During the period in 2021 between Trump's loss to Biden and Biden's transition into the White House and the Presidency, we, in the United States, were living in a postmodern moment of ontological rupture in which the continuation of democratic process was in doubt. As of this writing, Trump has still refused to admit that he lost to Biden, and continues to produce what, historically, has been termed, 'The Big Lie', in this case that Trump's election was stolen and that he, rather than Biden, was the victor.

There was an emptiness – a philosophical and pragmatic air pocket – in the west wing. The White House, itself, had become a Body without Organs. In his capacity for ruptured thetic statements and for his propensity for subverting systems of political convention and precedent, Trump qualifies as the first postmodern president perhaps since Truman, who dropped the bomb on Hiroshima ending the Second World War, and leading to a new awareness and concern with democracy and the nature of humanity.

Granting, for the moment, that Kristeva and Deleuze employ different frameworks for their work – Kristeva being a Lacanian, drawing from a psychoanalytic tradition, and DG ascribing an anti-oedipal schizo-analytic approach seeking other discourses as well as, and possibly apart from, the holy trinity of mother, father and son by which to access the human psyche – both Kristeva and DG suggest a similar structure in the chora of Plato's *Timaeus*.

Kristeva borrows the term chora from Plato, and describes it as something that, 'can be designated and regulated, [but] can never be definitively posited: as a result, one can situate the *khôra* and, if necessary, lend it a topology, but one can never give it axiomatic form' (*Revolution in Poetic Language*, 26)'.

The Kristevan reconceptualization of Plato's chora is the Oedipal psychoanalytic articulation of DG's schizo-analytic body without organs. Deleuze and Guattari use the term 'Body without Organs', which they describe as an empty surface, much like a piece of paper, that receives inscription and, as a result, conforms to the desires of those machines that attach themselves to it. One cannot simply have machines floating in nothingness any more than one can define something without language or words or a medium that will hold them in a position that can be called context. The body without organs lends itself a non-space of contextuality. Body without Organs, similarly to the chora, under Kristeva's understanding of the term, can also never be posited. One may lend the body without organs a topology, but, again like the chora, one can never give it axiomatic form.

Unlike the Kristevan chora, DG's body without organs exists outside the realm of particular discourse, theory and praxis. Deleuze does not dismiss the importance and even the validity of psychoanalysis so much as suggest the schizo also be aware of other discourses, etc. A body of organs, under this understanding could just as easily conform to psychoanalytic discourse as any other discourse – Marxism, Feminism, Capitalism, etc. The schizo-applicability of Deleuzean theory allows the BwO to be labelled under any number of different power formations – including that of schizophrenic capitalism during the tenure of a schizo president.

Trump's refusal both to leave office and to do any of the work required of the office resulted in an emptiness – a philosophical and pragmatic air pocket – in the west wing. This pocket is emblematic of Trump as the first postmodern president since Truman.

Though some might call it hyperbolic to compare Truman's dropping of a nuclear bomb on Japan to Trump's refusal to concede the presidency, Trump's refusal nonetheless ruptures the smooth transition of power – and thus political ideology – enjoyed traditionally between changes in administration. The concrete result of this refusal – Trump's truculence in eviscerating needed laws and departments, and his refusal to honor presidential tradition – is that the United States was without a leader. The philosophical result is that our political system, based on precedent, faced an unprecedented (and un-presidented) situation in which there was *neither* an arborescent transition based on law and precedent *nor*, a space for a rhizomal realm of potentiality (after the Kristevan *chora*) by which to reconstruct and reaffirm the constitutionally-expressed powers of governance through which we had been keeping our republic.

Politics – pandemic – president

Within the United States' two-party system, each political party is a machine that produces the desire to spread its own political ideology and political meaning while undermining that of its opponent. To one degree or another, American two-party politics has always tended toward partisan Hegelianism – positing the responsibility and the blame with the other party. This is the fault of neither party but rather results from an institutionalized ideological dialectic. Likewise, politics is an activity of presentation, positioning and persuasion rather than of monolithic truth. The fact that truth has to be qualified as 'monolithic', as opposed to having an alternative, is indication of the power of authoritarian discourse to re-code – as per the 'alternative facts' (facts asserted by Trump in opposition to either the media or the democrats) and 'fake news' (any news item that showed Trump and his administration in an unfavourable light), terms that gained widespread currency during the Trump Presidency and have all but disappeared with the start of Joe Biden's presidency in January of 2021. Of course, this is most likely due to Trump's twitter and Facebook and other social media accounts being suspended after he was tied to the attempted insurrection at the Capital Building on 6 January. 'Alternative facts' and 'fake news' are right-wing Trumpist terms, despite the fact that the media have co-opted them.

Both Democratic and Republican parties function as machines of political desire. For the sake both of historical accuracy and convenience, however, focus here is on the Trump political desiring machine as the hegemonic force present during the Covid pandemic as well as the dominant producer of hegemonic ideology and policy. The Trump Whitehouse both produced and enforced the economic, domestic and foreign policies governing the United States' response to the Covid pandemic and was behind the closing and the opening of national borders, in part following political directive, but more often reflecting the capitalist tendency not to recognize national boundaries. Where Democrats are seen to open borders and pay less attention to the open boundaries of big business in creating policy, Republicans in recent decades have tended to emphasize border security while at the same time loosening of national boundaries of other countries for the sake of its own benefit in international trade.

Virus – pathology and analogy

A virus is an infective agent that can only replicate within a host organism (https://www.nature.com/scitable/definition/virus-308/). A virus attaches to a particularly configured receptor on a cell's surface and is thereby able to enter the cell and to deposit genetic material that then combines with the cell's own genetic material in order to replicate itself. These replicated viruses are then deposited outside of the cell where they proceed to find other cells to continue the process of replication. The body then produces white blood cells to fight the onslaught of the replicating virus, which results in the body becoming sick and symptomatic. In the case of COVID-19, the lungs and the various mucous membranes of the body fill with a mixture of dead white blood cells and replicated viruses that the body then expels into the air, through coughing, sneezing, etc. The expelled viruses then float through the air, perhaps entering another body containing cells with the necessary receptors, and the process of infection and replication continues. The virus machine must attach to a compatible host machine, or cell, in order to synthesize a replication of itself. This synthesis most closely resembles the connective form, in that it produces an undifferentiated unity of product and process. The virus machine produces viruses. (That which we call the sickness, or the symptoms that the body produces in fighting the replication of viruses, is different from, and outside of, the production process of the virus itself.)

Analogies abound. Language is a virus. Culture is a virus. Ideas and ideation are viruses. Anything that uses a host to replicate and spread beyond that host into other hosts is a virus. An essay is a virus because it uses existing commentary and information to form its own body which then spreads through language to the brain which replicates it either in speaking or in writing perhaps producing mutations, new viral forms.

The virus, as with the analysis-code of an essay, is an assemblage that faces a body without organs. As a virus, analysis seeks to attach itself to the machine it analyses, so as to replicate that machine – that book, that other essay – with the materials of that essay, yet reproduced, or 'replicated' in its own terms, to conform to its own make-up and, in a sense, its own filter. This is much the same as what happens in reader response criticism – and what was always already there in any code of analysis aimed at sensical conclusions.

For Barthes, writing is the machine that destroys the author by de-theologizing him and the monolithic interpretation the author, as supreme authority has recognized him from pre-modern times.

> The reader is the space on which all the quotations that make up a writing are inscribed without any of them being lost; a text's unity lies not in its origin but in

> its destination. Yet this destination cannot any longer be personal: the reader is without history, biography, psychology; he is simply that someone who holds together in a single field all the traces by which the written text is constituted (The Death of the Author).

Yet, the reader is not, ultimately, a body without organs, despite Barthes' characterization of him as 'simply that someone who holds together in a single field all the traces by which the written text is constituted'. He is not 'simply' a memory bank devoid of analytical powers – and here, one imagines a person with an eidetic memory who retains information without processing it. But the careful reader will observe, rightly, that Barthes has already expanded upon this characterization when he states that the reader 'is someone who understands each word in its duplicity, and understands further, one might say, the very deafness of the characters speaking in front of him' (6). The reader, for Barthes, also produces – qualifying him as a machine, under Deleuze's definition – the canon and the acceptance and circulation of the text, as well as its critical corpus, among other things.

It happens the other way around, too. While analysis is certainly a machine that, as a virus, seeks to use the material of another machine to replicate itself – or versions, interpretations – of itself, so is the essay a viral machine that produces the raw materials for the analysis virus.

In the production of a rhizome, there is also implied the production of multiplicity and, therefore, diverse potentiality. When facing the body without organs, which it always has the potential of doing – as the facing of the assemblage to the body without organs *is* the manifestation of the potentiality of potential – the rhizomal network may appear *in potential* as the arrangement of roots reaching out from the arborescent. When in contact with the BwO, the 'points of contact' inscribed by the arborescent form a series of marks (each with signification, content, etc.) that may form a rhizomal network of multiply potential pathways and connections.

'Trump' is the arborescent system of desiring flow of all syntheses the name has signified or may come to signify under the various realms of politics, economics, hegemony, etc. 'Trump' always already contains a system of branches and roots, not all of which might be immediately visible until the rhizomal pattern of connections spoken of in the previous paragraph is connected. For this reason, the presence and power and connectivity of 'Trump' may, on the one hand, not be thoroughly accessible, and may, on the other, seem completely invisible and without cause or history (hence the tendency of pundits to define Trump as a sui generis phenomenon). Yet the visibility of Trump arises once the potential rhizomal network inscribes itself upon a suitable body without organs which may then be 'read' and analysed.

The political machine makes manifest political ideology and political meaning while at the same time both denying that is doing so and blaming the other side for doing it exclusively. Both democratic and republican parties function in this way as desiring machines – in this case, as machines of political desire. However, as Covid and the pandemic occurred during the Republican Trump administration – a political machine was recognized that differed markedly from both conventional Republican Conservatism and led to the possibility of the Republican party breaking into two parts – the traditional republican party, and for lack of a better name, the Trump party, or Trumpism. Trumpism inscribed within republicanism, and fuelled by a republican senate, was the dominant producer of hegemonic ideology during the pandemic. The Trump Whitehouse both produced enforced economic domestic and foreign policy during this period, behind the United States' response to the world stage on which the Covid pandemic was playing out. Trumpism was behind the closing and the opening of national borders, in part following political directive, but more often reflecting the Capitalist refusal of boundaries spoken about by Deleuze.

Desirability, jouissance and a few instances of Trumpian schizo-narrative

Before sending this essay machine off to synthesize with other machines in the ever non-complete work of desiring production, it's appropriate to infuse a bit of jouissance, as mentioned earlier, by presenting a few components of the Trumpian schizo-narrative that may fuel future schizo-analytic machines of desiring. This list of components will not serve as a conclusion for this essay – which is appropriate, because essays do not conclude; they simply make suggestions for future inquiry once the subject itself is processed and schizo-analytic desiring is produced.

A small, yet potentially overwhelming list of components of Trumpian schizo-narrativity

Trump is not Trump.

Trump is the label for an array of discourses and desiring machines that coalesce, potentially, in a rhizomal network whose actual centre is ever deferred. Trump resists definition and discourse. The discourse of Trump is ever-shifting, ever deferring, ever displacing, ever re-appropriating, ever exchanging, ever assigning and reassigning value.

The Trump name is not Trump, nor are the holdings of Trump, nor those centres of business that bear the Trump name, the belongings of Trump. The name Trump on a building does not refer to Trump, nor even to the Trump organization, although the latter is closer than the former.

This is no more unusual than the realization that the signifier is not the signified. Our names label us, but we may change them without necessarily affecting material change of our history, our psyche and our history. And yet, in the case of Trump, primarily because of a capitalist identity, we have a confusion – a schizo-affective interaction between Trump the signifier and Trump the signified – that must continually be reproduced in order for Trump in any manifestation to continue to exist.

Trump is a mode of production, the product of which is in continual flux, continual instability. Trump is a mode of production narrative, the product of which is Trump in various ideations and with various narratives.

Trump is the producer of alternative facts as well as the context for their acceptance among his followers. Trump is both medium and message.

The content of Trump is always another Trump.

The additional labelling of 'president' further complicates, for President is a title, and a position, assumed by the holder of the office.

Trump was always already there, and removing him does nothing to prevent his return.[1]

Note

1 With regard to the question of President Trump's rise to power, senior foreign correspondent, Adam E. Gallagher has the following to say: 'It strikes me that the whole Trump fiasco is the culmination of the two trends. Not only is Trump the raw, unbridled result of years of racist/nationalist/ individualist/militaristic GOP policy, but also the repulsive outgrowth of the dynamics of celebrity and Internet culture. Like pretty much everyone I know, I initially dismissed Trump's candidacy, but after this bizarre year and a half long spectacle it makes a lot more sense. Frankly, I know a lot of people that earnestly share Trump's racist worldview and think "businessmen" are a special breed of human with advanced intellectual capabilities [. . .] Trump is also the first true Internet/Reality TV candidate. He's only able to regurgitate soundbites and is capable of saying *literally* anything extemporaneously, which is part of the allure of both Reality TV and Trump. We've been conditioned by our entertainment outlets to expect quick, pithy, exciting moments; Trump provides that along with the catharsis of scapegoating whoever his audience needs to hate at that particular moment. As I wrote for ToM earlier this year, "The real story here – what Trump's risible and horrific place in American politics truly reveals – is that a large swathe of Americans are deeply, deeply uninformed." That was my nice way of saying that a lot of Americans are stupid.' ('Is Trump Sui Generis?' Tropics of Meta, 24 October 2016. https://tropicsofmeta.com/2016/10/24/is-trump-sui-generis/). We shall see in 2022, and perhaps 2024, whether Americans are any more well-informed or, as the case may be, any less stupid.

References

Barthes, Roland. 'The Death of the Author' in *Image, Music, Text* (S. Heath, Trans. and Ed.). London: HarperCollins, 1977, 142–148.

Deleuze, Gilles, and Guattari, F. L. *The Desiring Machines*. Minneapolis, MN: University of Minnesota Press, 1972.

Deleuze, Gilles, and Guattari, F. L. *Anti-Oedipus: Capitalism and Schizophrenia*. Minneapolis: University of Minnesota Press, 1983.

Deleuze, Gilles, and Guattari, F. L. *A Thousand Plateaus: Capitalism and Schizophrenia* (B. Massumi, Trans.). Minneapolis, MN: University of Minnesota Press, 1987.

Deleuze, Gilles, and Guattari, F. L. 'Introduction: Rhizome', in *A Thousand Plateaus: Capitalism and Schizophrenia* (B. Massumi, Trans.). Minneapolis, MN: University of Minnesota Press, 1987.

Kristeva, Julia. *Revolution in Poetic Language*. New York: Columbia University Press, 1984.

Plato. *Plato in Twelve Volumes*, Vol. 9 (W. R. M. Lamb, Trans.). Cambridge, MA, Harvard University Press; London, William Heinemann, 1925.

8

Regimes of Exclusion and Control: Politics of Modern Space and Its Role in the Immunization and Pandemics

Emine Görgül

Introduction

As we have been witnessing, with the COVID-19 outbreak in Spring 2020, the third decade of the new millennium began with the fundamental re-questioning of our contemporary life and its existential qualities. This novel condition not only cogitated the comfort zone of the civilized, biologically enhanced and technologically over-equipped human being but also mapped the interval as a fall in the history of modern times. As has been declared, ever since the aftermath of the Second World War, this new threat emerged as an unpredictable and fatal situation, occurring beyond the reign of current biotechnologies and governments' protective reflexes (BBC 2021). So, with the contagious spread of the virus, the modern liberal world hit the limits of liberty and the elusive utopia of democracy and equality, while at the same time we also encountered the strict reality of *regimes of exclusion and control*, whereas the post-war welfare state shifted into authoritarian ones, neglecting transnational identities.

As this novel invisible enemy immured us into our modern caves, the processes of *stratification*, *re-territorialization* and *interiorization* became the dominant acts within the urban realm to maintain the sanitization, isolation and surveillance during the struggle against the pandemic. Reciprocally, these *force majeure* actions were globally adopted by governments, so that extreme measures of surveillance and control were manifested: such as closing down the borders, prohibiting the flows, coding and tracing citizens for transnational insulation at the end. Thus, the infected citizen and the infected space became the other for the system, to be excluded and combatted. As a consequence, the State occurred as the sovereign power in the processes of deterritorialization of the invisible enemy, activating itself as a defence force, the immunity system of society.

On the other hand, Latour (1993) advocates that the cycles of the outbreak, inclusion and control of epidemics, and their transformative capacities were the fundamental phases in the modern way of conceptualizing our life. To validate his hypothesis, Latour focuses on the scientific interventions of nineteenth-century Europe and prioritizes the inventions in medicine for enhancing immunity systems. He addresses the interval as the climax of a two-fold immunization process. On one side, the immunized body of the citizen against the pathogens serves in the constitution of the community's collective body. And on the other, this collective body of the community becomes the State's immunity mechanism, defending its persistence and sovereignty against any threat or the enemy. Hand in hand with Latour's reading of intertwined relations among medicine, bureaucracy and state power, Esposito (2013) also discusses the notion of immunization in the realm of the community as well as its political and economic resemblances. He emphasizes that immunity arises as a reflex mechanism that operates in a regulatory order via diverse and *in situ* decision-making and negotiating processes.

In this sense, departing from Latour's and Esposito's take on immunity as a process rather than a status, then the act of immunization could be claimed as an agency, enhancing the individual and collective body of the community through diverse inter-connected processes. More specifically, from a Deleuzoguattarian perspective, this intertwined procedure could be interpreted as a *machinic assemblage* either through ways and means of inoculation and vaccine or through treatment protocols and their spatiality for care and cure. However, for the desperate cases where stratification and isolation are obliged, then the *disjunctive synthesis* becomes an alternative process in the spatio-political planning to maintain surveillance and control of the other.

So, regarding the agency of both the human body and the architectural space in the constitution of immunity and strength against the visible and the invisible enemies, this chapter aims to question the role of spatio-politics in the processes of immunization. It further aims to reveal how architecture reacts to the dialectics of humanitarian aid and authoritarian restriction in the two-fold reality of treatment and segregation, inclusion and control. Within this scope, the impacts of immunology and biopolitics in the place-making practices during the last hundred years of modernization arise as the topics to be discussed. In this way, the chapter validates its essential hypothesis that, similar to medicine and biology, architecture has been a crucial component and a critical player in immunization and biopolitics. It tacitly and directly acts and takes part in the State's war against the (in)visible enemy or any emerging threat while re-territorializing its power through building its regimes of either care, cure and augmentation or exclusion, insulation and control both during the pandemics and in the wider processes of immunization. Accordingly, the notions of control, surveillance, stratification, decontamination, triage, segregation and isolation are also opened into a discussion together with their counter-terms like resilience, solidarity, connectedness or anarchy and decay on behalf of place-making practices.

The chapter initially reveals the notion of immunity from diverse aspects of biology, politics and biopolitics. Then, in the following parts, the role of – modern – architecture and its designated spaces – the invented typologies – of treatment and isolation are discussed reciprocally with the assembling forces, the behaviours of stratification, and the regimes of exclusion and control. The chapter concludes its debate by questioning the possibility of two contradicting lines of flights as the ultimate tracks in the immunization: autotoxicus or autopoiesis.

Immunology, body and biopolitics

Before rising to the degree of a pandemic, on the very initial level any particular disease occurs through the *assembling* properties of both the contaminated body (the host) and the newly emerging pathogen (the agent) (Principles of Epidemiology 2012, 1–72). The biological definition of *pathogen* addresses 'a bacterium, virus, or another microorganism that can cause disease' (Merriam-Webster n.d.). However, from a broader interpretation of the term, it also refers to the agency of an – infectious – medium, that causes a change. This single change, or series of changes, differentiates the former condition of meta-stability within the system by replacing it with sequential processes of transformation. So, the contagiousness appears as an unsolidified, transitive and momentary becoming within the vectorial flow of causative agencies. On the other hand, the condition of being contaminated is also defined as an interruption in the flow, relatively a sedimentation, indicating the status of being infected. The moment of being contaminated further becomes a threshold of potential discriminative processes or excluding attempts, as the specific causative agent, the unknown outsider, occurs as a potential threat to the system, or the immunity.

In biological terms, immunity is defined as the system protecting the organism by 'having or producing bodies of defense (antibodies) capable of reacting with a specific agency (antigen)' (Merriam-Webster n.d.). It is almost conceived 'as a military apparatus' being assigned to 'conserve[e], preserv[e], and observ[e] the self against foreign intruders' (Bird and Short 2017, 304). These defensive capacities further constitute a paradigm for the reflexive or hegemonic interpretations of the immunity system. Doubtless, this broadening interpretation of the immunity paradigm enables it to move beyond the field of biology, towards social, political and spatial realms, while assigning a decisive role to it in the constitution of our contemporary life.

The conceptualization of immunity and life is recognized as the turning point in the organization of modern life and society. The invention of modern biology in the nineteenth century is acknowledged as a starting point in defining novel inquiries of originality (Saidel 2014). According to Foucault, the transfiguring formulation of life grounds itself in the dissociation from earlier definitions of life formats (*bios*) from the natural environment (*Zoe*), on behalf of protecting the life from death via developing a novel territorial or conditional reality (Foucault 2008; Saidel 2014). This fundamental shift from the former inquiries of ancient times into the domination of the immunity paradigm addresses the origins of modern life. So, unlike emerging in a milieu of existence naturally open to any vectors or agents to be connected, the modern format of life exists firmly in the milieu that is protected by the immunity that controls and defines itself. Yet, the protective role of immunity not only maintains the continuity of the organism's life or the individual, but also the community itself; whereas the vectorial flow of a causative agent to the other organism in the comity might be blocked. Thus, the status of being alive prioritizes the role of immunity in the formation of the community, so the modern life (Esposito 2013). In this respect, any possibility of acquired immunity versus the natural one constituted the essence of modernization and biopolitics, where the immunization 'becomes a strategic decision' defining the sustainability, sovereignty and liberty of the community (Saidel 2014, 113).

Reciprocally, referring to the diseases and infections of the eighteenth and nineteenth centuries, in his work *The Pasteurization of France*, Latour (1993) discusses these intertwined connections of individual and communal immunity reflexes concerning the systems of healing and bureaucracy. Latour begins developing his argument by highlighting two cases: the drastic defeat of Napoleon's army on the battlefield and – a century later – the emancipating scientific victory of Pasteur with his invention of vaccination against the invisible enemy of microbes. He draws the connections between the immunization of the body and the persistence of State power through the agency of citizens' embodiment and medicine. Similar to Esposito's definition of immunity to the community in the frame of biopolitics, while transforming into a homogenized and stratified entity of State power, the agency of the enhanced embodiment of the citizens becomes a medium and the active power of combat on behalf of the State. More specifically, as medical and pharmaceutical procedures de-territorialize the milieu of existence for the microbes, viruses and bacteria, the power of the State re-territorializes both the citizen and the territorial sovereignty through the agency of the attained collective immunity. So, the intertwined connection of State power and control, war and medicine are all reflected and constituted via gradual enhancement of citizens' immunity, and this establishes the essence of modern society over the last few hundred years.

This positivist certainty of attaining success in the augmentation of the individual and the collective embodiment positions agency or mediation at the centre of discussion. Referring to the notion of technology (*techné*), Esposito similarly affirms its inevitable presence in attaining the acquired level of immunity, where technology operates as a completer to fulfil the lacking capacities of the human (Esposito 2008). This critical and constructive role of technology not only re-affirms the dignity between the ancient way of living and modern life but also provides the interconnection among modern life and politics, the hegemonic condition of immunity and biology, biopolitics and powers of sovereignty, and the persistence of the state.

In the same way, we can think of various technologies with diverse fields and levels of competence serving the main goal of immunity and related policies. In other words, beyond the agency of medical and pharmaceutical technologies, macro-technologies of space and politics also operate as the mediums for collective immunity through the diverse processes of interiorization, exclusion or control. While asking '[w]hat is immunization, if not a progressive interiorization of an outside?', Esposito not only accepts all the bodies inside the threshold as equivalent and collectively enfolding similar conditions of immunity, but he also spatializes the notion in between the stable side of the controlled interior and the uncontrolled outside. Indeed, inquiries of immunization are also associated with technologies of place-making, while calling architecture and space into charge, as well as interrogating Foucaultian biopolitics at the same time. So, recalling Hardt and Negri's (2000) emphasis on the world with no more outside, we no longer claim a territorial condition excluded from the hegemony of the immunity paradigm, and its definite stratification processes for attaining the contemporary condition of modern society.

Architecture and disease: immunization as an assemblage to cure and enhance

The bond between health and space has a long history, dating back to ancient times. As Colomina (2011) highlights, '[f]or as long as we remember, or for as long as history remembers, architecture has followed medicine', whereas the reverse of the equilibrium could also be claimed. In this respect, we have observed not only the apparent connection between illness, treatment and architecture but also the concrete outcomes of their interactions. These outcomes occurred both on the level of knowledge and the constitution of space, on behalf of maintaining healthier environments in the domestic and the public realm. The birth of novel typologies like hospitals and specialized treatment centres such as sanatoriums was also the result of these two-fold interactions.

Historically, the notorious architect of ancient times Vitruvius appeared as the initial source in western architectural history, mentioning the linkages between health and architecture, and their account of the constitution of healthier environments (Bruno 1997). So, quoting from Cesariano's (1521) translation of Vitruvius' *De Architectura* – Ten Books on Architecture (first-century BC) 'Healthfulness being their [architects'] chief object'; Colomina claims that Vitruvius further proposed a trans-disciplinary aspect, through insisting on a cross-pollination among architecture and medicine education (Colomina 2019). In this way, the body of architectural knowledge would be boosted with the injection of another expertise – medicine – to create superior spaces for enhancing the immunity of the body of the human and the architectural space.

On the other hand, though Vitruvius mostly refers to the human embodiment as a healthy, stiff, durable and profound one at the very centre of the cosmos, the possibility of feeling not well, sick, even unhealthy, was also the reality for ancient societies. Roman *Asklepios* emerged as the initial architectural typology for health in Ancient times, while acting as treatment centres for both physical and mental health with a holistic aspect (Walton 1894). They were constructed on both sides of the Aegean Sea and gradually institutionalized by the fourth century BC (Walton 1894). Roman *Asklepios* were not only the spatial precursors of modern hospitals by introducing genuine spatial organizations such as preliminary implementations of the ward system, but also occurred as the founding epicentres of modern medicine (Bayatlı 1947). Eminent figures of modern medicine such as Hippocrates also experimented with these medical practices (Walton 1894). As is acknowledged, the Roman *Asklepios* were mostly dedicated to the treatment of soldiers, where various techniques referring to material and immaterial assemblages of body and medicine were deployed: such as dream and inducement therapies, treatments based on nutrition and mineral water intake, engagement with nature and bodily exercises as well as surgeries (Walton 1894).

Despite the promotion of good health in Antiquity from the multiple perspectives of philosophy, architecture and medicine, the emergence of the plague epidemic by the end of the Medieval Age and its consequences were decisive in the reconfiguration of our perception of the body. The severity of the disease triggered the inquiries of cure and immunization processes as well as their associating spatiality. Thus, the former paradigm of the centrality of the human condition – like it was in the depictions of Vitruvian man – and healthiness of the body shifted into a vulnerable, imperfect and unhealthy embodiment existing in a peripheral condition while generating a novel set of knowledge and reality (Healy 2006). In this respect, the imperfect body was decentralized from the centre of the universe; however, based on the life and the vulnerability of the human, the guarding eye of immunity, cure and control was centralized into the spatiality.

Recalling the earlier discussions on the conceptualization of modern life and immunity and the interiorization as a reterritorialization process of the milieu of existence, apparently, this translocation of the eye is also connected with our modernist conceptualization of immunity. Doubtless, the literal and figurative centralization of the caring and controlling eye was performed through the revolutionary design of hospitals in the eighteenth century (Wagenaar 2020). These advancements further signified a critical turn in the deployment of technologies of place-making for immunization against diseases. In this respect, even before Bentham's (1995) invention of the *panopticon* in 1791 (Figure 8.1) – the archetypical model of the surveillance mechanism by placing the invisible eye on the epicentre of the prison space for discipline and control – the modern hospital design in 1770s Paris introduced a further challenge in discussing the role of architecture and the place-making practices in the immunization processes.

As Wagenaar discusses, the architectural projects developed for the D'Hôtel Dieu Paris (Figure 8.2) from 1772–1788 were groundbreaking spatial interventions, positioning the centrality of immunity and treatment – for a healthier body – at the core of the contemporary hospital typology (Wagenaar 2020).

He further claims the design of the D'Hôtel Dieu was almost a *machinic phylum*, being generated to heal people, while 'liberating the hospital – and healthcare in general – from the constraints of religion, conventions, traditions and superstitions' (Wagenaar 2020, 38). In this way, the modern hospital of the eighteenth century addressed an evident split from its further perception and organizational structure. It was also claimed to perform innovative spatial mechanisms to heal the patients via integrating various sub-systems like ventilation, sewage and therapeutic environment.

In other words, this envisions the modern hospital as a *machinic phylum* consisting of diverse sub-systems operating for healing and immunization, bringing two intertwined notions of *connective synthesis* and *assemblage* into the discussion. On one side, all those functioning mechanical sub-systems of sanitation and treatment that were immersed in the architectural design of the hospital typology operated through a connective synthesis. Thus, resonating with Deleuze and Guattari's (1987) take on the productive content of the synthesis, and the integrated facilities of the diverse sub-systems as a novel unity, the emergence of eighteenth-century hospitals came into being as the specific case of producing a novel ecosystem, the modern milieus of treatment and care.

On the other hand, the evident bond among the assembling forces of medicine–architecture–disease and patient, as well as the connective properties of the healing spaces, were mapped during the tuberculosis epidemic in the twentieth century.

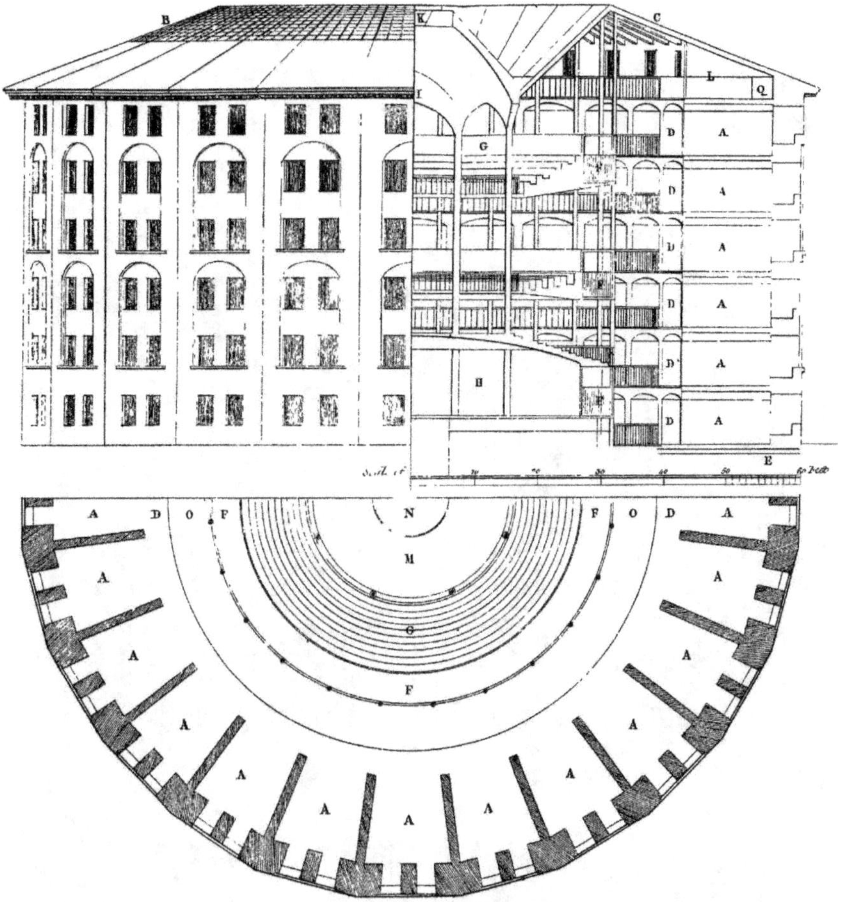

Figure 8.1 Plan of Jeremy Bentham's panopticon prison, drawn by Willey Reveley in 1791. Reproduced under a Creative Commons Attribution-Share Alike 4.0 International license. https://commons.wikimedia.org/wiki/File:Plan_of_Jeremy_Bentham%27s_panopticon_prison,_drawn_by_Willey_Reveley_in_1791.jpg

Referring to the earlier discussion on the use of technology in the enhancement of immunity and its acquired level in the community, the invention of sanatorium typology in the last century addressed another significant interval in re-examining the mediocracy role and capacities of the modern architectural embodiment of healthcare spaces. As Aalto (1956) states, '[t]he main purpose of the [sanatorium] building is to function as a medical instrument' (Schildt 1994; Colomina 2019, 65), almost an apparatus to cure the infected body of the patient with its innovatively designed spatial embodiment.[1] As Colomina highlights, disease enabled architecture to practise a more radical solution to accommodate the excessive amount of sunlight and fresh air needed to eradicate it (Colomina 2019, 63). On one side, facades became more transparent

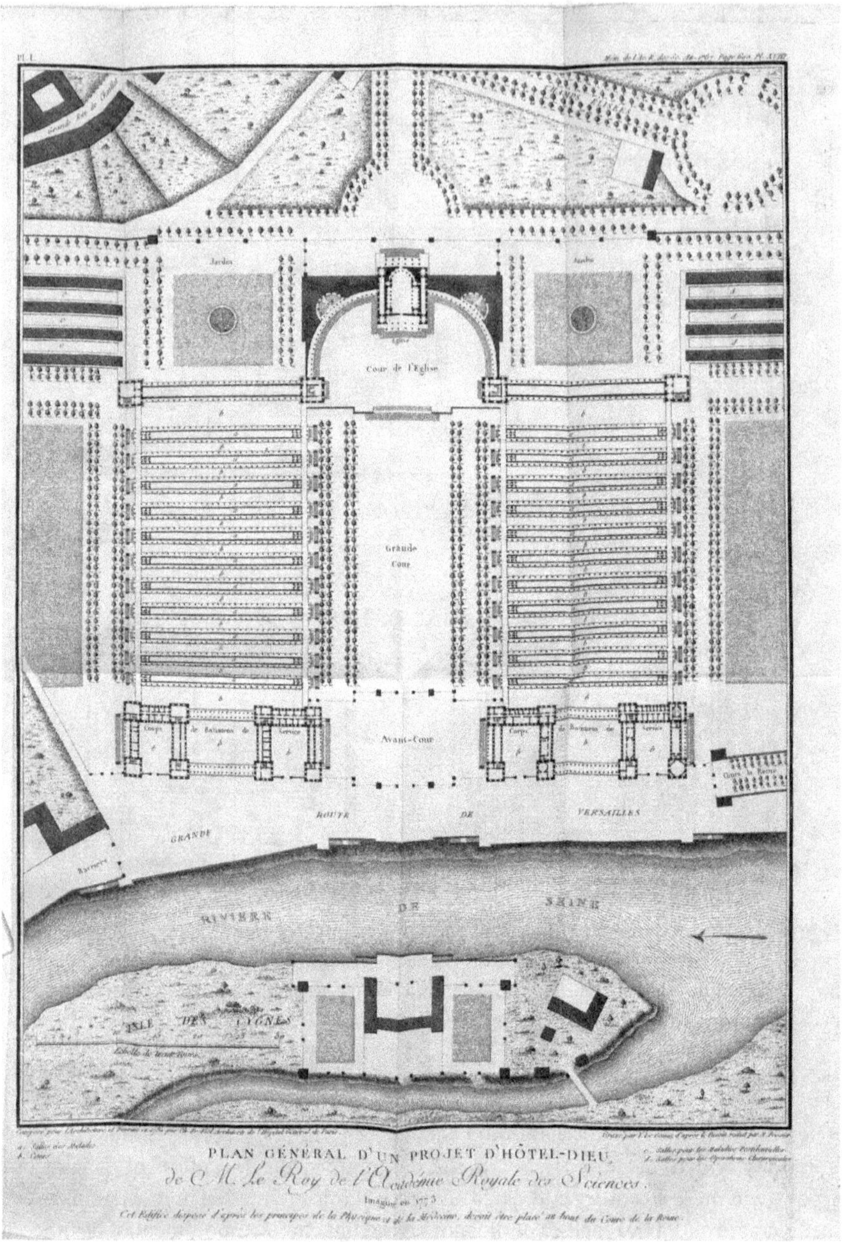

Figure 8.2 General plan of a new Hôtel-Dieu at Chaillot district, by architect Charles-François Viel based on an idea by Jean-Baptiste Le Roy, 1787, Paris. Reproduced under a Creative Commons Attribution-Share Alike 4.0 International license. https://commons.wikimedia.org/wiki/File:Plan_General_d%27un_Projet_d%27Hotel-Dieu,_1787_-_Cornell_University_Library.tif

with their glazed skins to take the maximum amount of sunlight and fresh air, and on the other, long and generous balconies were attached to the facades for longer outdoor sunbathing treatments. So, different from the eighteenth-century hospitals, the twentieth-century sanatorium design introduced the machinic assemblages among the sunlight, the infected body of the patient, and the striped architectural embodiment as its groundbreaking novelty.

Referring to Esposito's inquiries on interiorization, immunization and community, the sanatoriums could be considered the ultimate examples of modern architecture responding to a condition of epidemic and disease. So, with the maximum interiorization of macro-ecological vectors, immunization becomes an assemblage of negotiation among the heterogeneous elements into a productive entity for the collective immunity. In other words, the interaction between architecture and disease has been affirmed through the connective synthesis of spaces for treatment and care, which came into being through the multi-fold genesis of material, immaterial and biological formations (Deleuze and Guattari 1987).

Architecture and control: immunization as a disjunction to isolate and segregate

Referring to Hardt and Negri's (2000) take on the world with no more outside, and the fact that the lack of a territorial condition was excluded from the hegemony of the immunity paradigm, the process of interiorization not only leads towards care and cure in terms of enhancing the collective body but also re-folds upon itself to demark the unimmunized ones. In other words, a process of re-interiorization emerges to maintain the persistence of the collective immunity, where the spatial mechanisms of this double interiority emerge as the mechanisms of disjunction. Thus, unlike the connective synthesis of space and immunization in the cure and care, the *disjunctive synthesis* of spatial relations for re-interiorization leads towards the augmentation of authoritarian power of immunity, via providing isolation, exclusion and control of the bodies that are assigned already as the other.

Deleuze and Guattari (1987) explain the disjunction as the production of differences in the sense of accommodating the multiple syntheses of 'either . . . or' for the productive ways of acknowledging the existential qualities. In other words, for Deleuze and Guattari, the multitude of differences in the disjunctive synthesis enfolds inclusive and affirmative content rather than exclusive and restrictive. However, in the processes of double interiorization, for attaining the ultimate immunity, the possible emergence of difference arises as the potential threat to be isolated and discarded from the system.

The characteristics of otherness are mostly defined as a condition or state of being different from and alien to the social identity of a person and the identity of the self (Miller 2008). Referring to Foucault (1987), with the advent of modernity, the other is accepted as the un-immunized one: those such as criminals, the physiologically or mentally disordered, the ethically deteriorated, which have also been marked as the ones to be excluded from society in terms of maintaining order and the collective immunity. So, as Foucault argues, the spatial interfaces of prisons, asylums or, at the extreme end, detention camps emerge as spatial patterns in strictly classifying and confining the ones that are already discarded.

Tracing back in history, probably the myth of the labyrinth emerges as the most fundamental archetypical definition of this double interiority, where the extreme stratification of the confined is spatially constituted (Hahn 2013). Thus, as in the case of architect Daedalus' invention of the labyrinth space, where the Minotaur–the other body is kept, the *striated space* of the labyrinth operates as an *apparatus of capture*. So, the mechanisms of confinement propose the immobility of the detained; they also present controlled environments and inescapable spatialities of repression that consist of molar structures of unified interiorities. In this respect, while resonating with the homogenized characteristic of the enclosure, Giovanni Battista Piranesi's notorious images from the eighteenth century of the fictive atmospheric drawings of prisons – *carceri* (Pinto and Pinto 2016) – emerge as remarkable representations that visualize the imperceptible structure of their labyrinthine interiors (Thompson 2003; Figure 8.3).

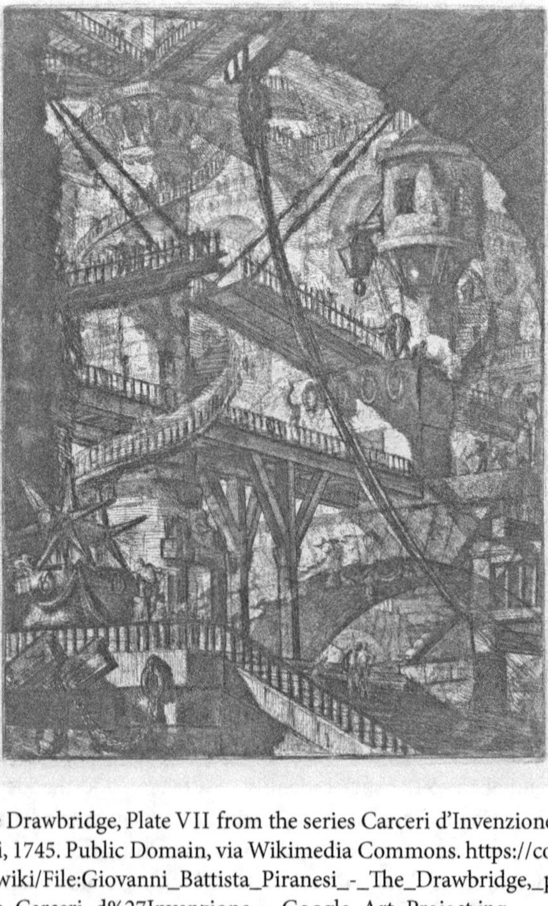

Figure 8.3 'The Drawbridge, Plate VII from the series Carceri d'Invenzione' by Giovanni Battista Piranesi, 1745. Public Domain, via Wikimedia Commons. https://commons.wikimedia.org/wiki/File:Giovanni_Battista_Piranesi_-_The_Drawbridge,_plate_VII_from_the_series_Carceri_d%27Invenzione_-_Google_Art_Project.jpg

Piranesi depicts the dark, vaulted crypt-like hostile spaces of no-man's-land, which also reflect strong impressions of the uncanny (Vidler 1992, 40). As Piransesian *carceris* unfold through eternity, without indicating any resemblance of scale or a spatial reference of differentiation, they also avoid conveying any hints about a feeling of neither a beginning nor an end. In addition, the strong sense of timelessness emerges as the prevalent perception across the images, where the viewer's confined gaze appears to be frozen within the dark interiors, together with the immense sensation of the static interiority of the prison that subliminally emphasizes the immobility.

Thus, imperceptibility, immobility and timelessness constitute the essential characteristics of these confining realms, which in the end become the actual spaces of oppression. Doubtless, in these spaces of oppression, the notion of *subjugation* becomes inevitable. Hence, these spaces are further associated with various means of power and sovereignty relations, together with the aforementioned frozen characteristics of time, causing submissive models of authoritarian spaces to arise (Stoner 2012, 9, 19). In other words, spaces of oppression emerge as *striated* spaces of *molar* structures where everything is defined, classified and homogenized in such a way that the autocratic power controls and assimilates it via the spatial relations of hegemony and power (Deleuze and Guattari, 1987).

Concluding remarks: towards an autopoietic or autotoxicus genesis of space

While defining the notion of existence or the concept of becoming, Deleuze and Guattari (1987) deploy both the notion of virus and the contagion to explain diverse means and ways of assemblage and transformation from the perspective of difference. They emphasize the notions of contagion and epidemics as ways of 'peopling, propagation, a becoming that is without ... a filiation or a hereditary production' almost in a similar fashion to battlefields and catastrophes (1987, 241). And referring to the example of the vampire, which does not filiate, but infects, they prioritize the heterogeneous characteristics of the assembling forces among the agent and the host and their un-natural participation towards forming a combination of an *interkingdom* (1987, 242).

So, winding back the spool to the vectorial flow of the contagious and the assembling properties of un-akin entities of a causative agent and the systematic embodiment, the recently formed organism of the *interkingdom* reshapes or outlines its conditions for an alternative immunity that leads towards its prospect epigenesis. According to Deleuze and Guattari in this *aparallel evolution*, like in the capacities of the viruses, the evolutionary trajectory 'take[s] a flight and move into entirely different species' (1987, 10). So, as they highlight the excluded potential of sedimentation or structural formation towards attaining an evolutional result; then the body of the *aparallel evolution* becomes the other to be transformed and to translocate itself until it is disconnected or unplugged one more time.

Yet, Deleuze and Guattari envision both contagion and viral encounters from an affirmative perspective, far from the *molar segmentary* of any defence mechanisms or processes of stratification. Thus, the immunity system is re-conceptualized no longer from 'a defensive and reactionary manner, but rather in a more tolerant manner' (Bird and Short 2017, 303). In this way, novel trajectories could be claimed towards affirming difference and heterogeneity within the system. Accordingly, two different lines of flight become applicable either in the frame of auto-immunity disorder or autopoiesis. On one side autopoiesis maintains adaptation towards continuity, whereas auto-immunity disorder leads to termination and collapse.

As Guerra-Filho (2014) highlights, autopoiesis and auto-immunity disorder emerge from each other, through their intertwined relations. As he calls into attention, the paradox of misbehaving immunity emerges from the 'legal autopoiesis ending up in auto-immunity' (21). He further emphasizes that '[a]uto-immunity is an aporia: the very thing that aims to protect us is the thing that destroys us' (Guerra-Filho 2014, 21). This is the condition that Protevi mentions when the negotiating powers of immunity can no longer communicate with the individual cell or the entire body, then it targets itself through 'assimilation or rejection and excretion' (Protevi 2001, 102). It is at this moment that the host becomes hostile to itself and targets actions against itself while paving the way to destruction.

Not surprisingly, architectural interventions once more provide concrete examples, through which the intertwined relations among the autopoiesis and auto-immunity disorder of the system could be dismantled in more detail. Significantly, the modern mass housing projects of the mid-twentieth century emerged as cases where immense interiorization processes of the post-war realm leads to auto-immunity disorders. As the States prioritized the sustainable development of the welfare policies and the comfort of the citizens, these mass-housing projects emerged as the main spatio-political mediums to stratify, sediment and immunize the society by creating akin environments. However, these extremely homogenized environments failed to control and suppress the possible trajectories for autopoietic lines of flight.

For instance, the case of Märkisches Viertel in West Berlin (Figure 8.4), in the mid-1960s, emerged as one of the key examples with its unusual epigenesis story. It was once designed as 'an expressive composition that embodies a will to art and sensible and not only mechanistic spatial order', then turns into a case of 'ugly architecture and bad planning' reflecting the totalitarian face of the State (Urban 2015, 180–181).

Recalling Negt and Kluge's take on public space and the transformation of the bourgeois public sphere into an inclusive one serving the majority, during the 1968 student protest in Berlin, the Märkisches Viertel appeared as the epicentre of radical activists like Ulrike Meinhof and her friends, acting more like a scene while reclaiming public space for agitation and anti-State propaganda (Urban 2015; Passmore 2011). The anonymity of the housing space and its inhabitants due to the over-stratification space further fuelled the inquiries of miscommunication and the weakening authority of the State. So, reverting this private space into a public one, initially, non-violent protests were performed with the use of diverse broadcasting technologies, video interviews or radio plays like *Bambule* (1970), where some of the activists later converted themselves into some underground factions (Wallace 2016). It was not only the result of the State's over interiorization at the Märkisches Viertel that enabled the auto-immunity disorder that empowered the opposition and resistance but also that of

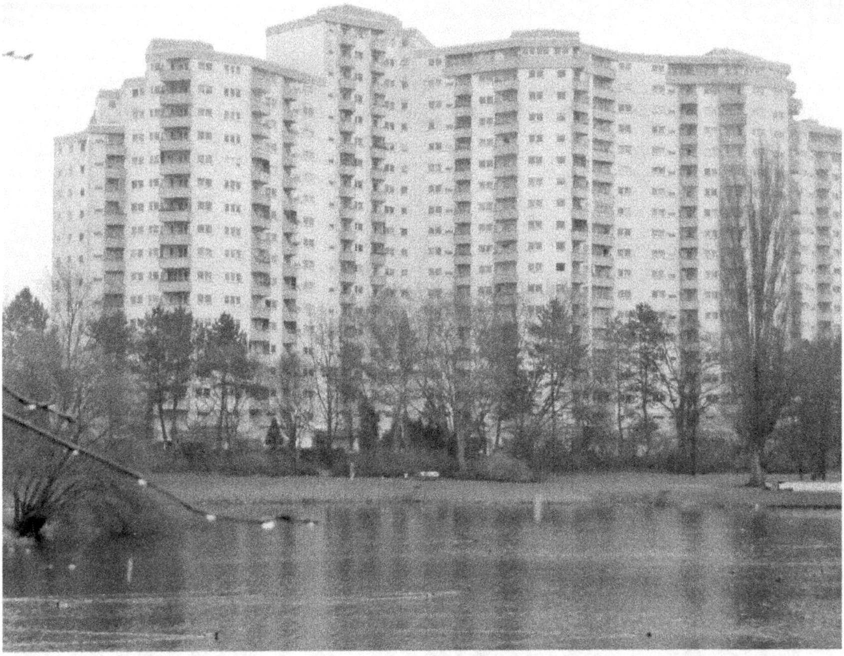

Figure 8.4 Märkisches Neighborhood, Residential Buildings by architects Werner Georg Heinrichs, Werner Düttmann, Oswald Mathias Ungers, René Gagès and Chen Kuen Lee, 1962–68, Berlin © Miriam Guterland, 2016. Reproduced under a Creative Commons Attribution-Share Alike 3.0 Unported license. https://commons.wikimedia.org/wiki/File:M%C3%A4rkisches_Viertel_Berlin_Archtitekt_Chen_Kuen_Lee.JPG

the *aparallel evolution* of the contagious assemblages of the users – significantly the Ulrike Meinhof's – and the space that broke the molar segmentary.

Nevertheless, the mid-twentieth-century housing project Pruitt-Igoe, in St Louis, Missouri, marks the end-point of how auto-immunity disorder was finalized by autotoxicus reactions, leading ultimately to a death drive (Figure 8.5). The ultimate biopolitical stratification of society based on race and class created an over-homogenized territorial condition so that, due to extreme conditions, immunity began to function against itself by harming the organism via violence and vandalism, in the end destroying everything.

To conclude: although the re-birth of the pandemic in the twenty-first century has reintroduced us to the spaces of quarantine and cure from the perspective of disease and immunity, the longer history of immunology and biopolitics openly declares its close collaboration with the regimes of control by also deploying spatial interventions as its fundamental tool. So, via diverse tactics of interiorization or exteriorization, the immunization aims to stratify the community to gain its maximum ruling power. Yet, referring to the connective and disjunctive capacities of the classification and

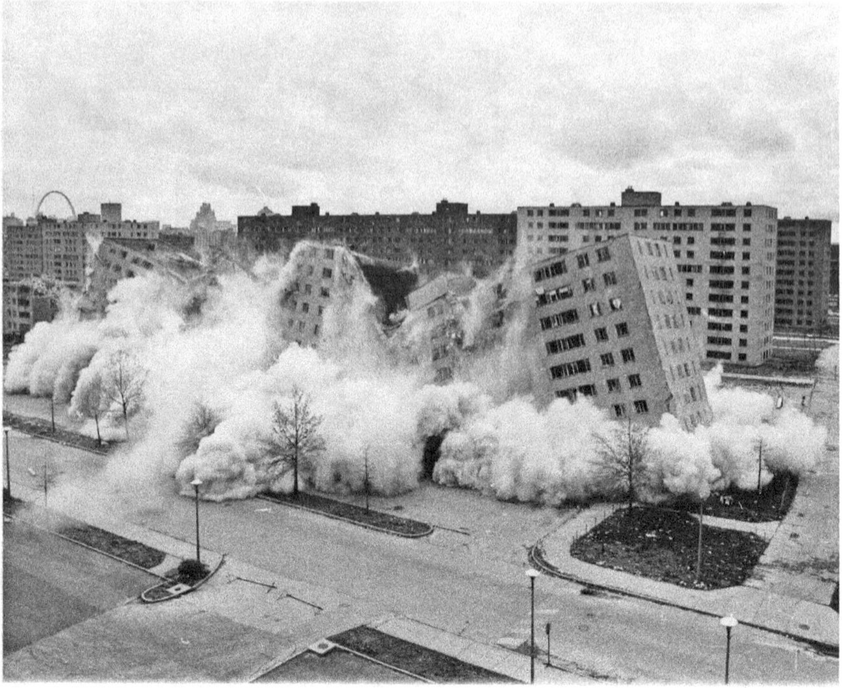

Figure 8.5 Destruction of Pruitt-Igoe housing Project on 21 April 1972. U.S. Department of Housing and Urban Development Office of Policy Development and Research. Wikimedia Commons, Public Domain. https://commons.wikimedia.org/wiki/File:Pruitt-Igoe-collapses.jpg

stratification, in the light of mutation there exist alternative paths throughout the system towards the refrain or towards the flight.

Note

1 Quoting from Schildt, Colomina refers to Aalto's lecture in Italy, about Paimio Sanatorium in 1956.

References

Bayatlı, O. (1947), *Bergama Tarihinde Asklepion* [Asklepion in Pergamon History] İzmir: Doğanlar Basımevi.

BBC (2021), 'Covid: 2020 Saw Most Excess Deaths Since World War Two', BBC, 12 January 2021. Available online: https://www.bbc.com/news/uk-55631693

Bentham, J. (1995), *The Panopticon Writings*, New York: Verso.

Bird, G., Short, J. (2017), 'Cultural and Biological Immunization: A Biopolitical Analysis of Immigration Apparatuses' in *Configurations*, Vol. 25, No. 3, Johns Hopkins University Press, pp. 301–326.

Bruno, L. C. (1997), 'De Architectura, Cesare Cesariano, Male Human Body, 1521' in *The Tradition of Technology: Landmarks of Western Technology in the Collections of the Library of Congress*, Washington, DC: Library of Congress

Colomina, B. (2011), 'Illness as Metaphor in Modern Architecture' in *Caring Culture: Art, Architecture, and Politics of Public Health*, A. Philips and M. Miessen (eds.) Berlin: Sternberg Press.

Colomina, B. (2019), *X-Ray Architecture*, Baden: Lars Müller Publishers.

Esposito, R. (2008), *Bíos: Biopolitics and Philosophy*, trans. Timothy Campbell, Minneapolis: University of Minnesota Press.

Esposito, R. (2013), *Terms of the Political: Community, Immunity, Biopolitics,* trans. Rhiannon Noel Welch, New York: Fordham University Press.

Foucault, M. (1987), *Mental Illness and Psychology.* M. Senellart (ed.), Berkeley: University of California Press.

Foucault, M. (2008), *The Birth of Biopolitics: Lectures at the College de France, 1978–79*, M. Senellart (ed.), New York: Palgrave McMillan.

Gilles, D., Guattari, F. (1983), *Anti-Oedipus: Capitalism and Schizophrenia*, Minneapolis: University of Minnesota Press.

Gilles, D., Guattari, F. (1987), *A Thousand Plateaus: Capitalism and Schizophrenia*, trans. Brian Massumi, Minneapolis: University of Minnesota Press.

Guerra-Filho, W. (2014), *Immunological Theory of Law*, LAP-Lambert Academic Publishing.

Hardt, M., Negri, A. (2000), *Empire*, Cambridge MA: Harvard University Press.

Hahn, J. (2013), *Labyrinth, The Shape of the Modern Mind: Kafka, Auster, Borges*, Wellesley College, Honors in Comparative Literature, Wellesley College Digital Scholarship and Archive. Retrieved from http://repository.wellesley.edu/cgi/viewcontent.cgi?article=1143&context=thesiscollection

Healy, P. (2006), 'The Stoical Body', in *The Body in Architecture*, Rotterdam: 010 Publishers, pp. 115–129.

Latour, B. (1993), *The Pasteurization of France,* trans. Alan Sheridan, John Law, Cambridge MA: Harvard University Press.

Merriam-Webster. (n.d.), Pathogen. In *Merriam-Webster.com dictionary.* Retrieved 28 November 2021, from https://www.merriam-webster.com/dictionary/pathogen

Miller, J. (2008). 'Otherness'. *The SAGE Encyclopedia of Qualitative Research Methods.* Thousand Oaks, CA: SAGE, pp. 588–591.

Passmore, L. (2011), *Ulrike Meinhof and the Red Army Faction: Performing Terrorism*, New York: Palgrave Macmillan.

Pinto, J. A., Pinto, M. (2016). *Rome City of the Soul.* New York: MLM Publication and Morgan Library and Museum.

Protevi, J. (2001), *Political Physics: Deleuze, Derrida, and the Body Politic*, London: Athlone Press.

Principles of Epidemiology in Public Health Practice: An Introduction to Applied Epidemiology and Biostatistics (2012), Self-Study Course SS197, U.S. Department of Health and Human Services, Atlanta: Centers for Disease Control and Prevention (CDC).

Saidel, M. I. (2014), 'Biopolitics and Its Paradoxes: An Approach to Life and Politics in R. Esposito', in *Rivista Lo Sugardo*, No. 15, pp. 109–131.

Schildt, G. (1994), *Alvar Aalto: The Complete Catalogue of Architecture, Design, and Arts*, trans. Timothy Binham, New York: Rizolli Minnesota Press.
Stoner, J. (2012), *Towards a Minor Architecture*. Cambridge: MIT Press.
Thompson, W. (2003), 'Giovanni Battista Piranesi (1720–1778)', in *Heilbrunn Timeline of Art History*. New York: Metropolitan Museum of Arts. Retrieved from http://www.metmuseum.org/toah/hd/pira/hd_pira.htm
Urban, F. (2015), 'The Märkisches Viertel in West-Berlin' in *Architecture and the Welfare State*, M. Swenarton, T. Avermaete, D. Van Heuvel (eds.), New York: Routledge, pp. 177–198.
Vidler, A. (1992), *Architectural Uncanny: Essays in the Modern Unhomely*, Cambridge: MIT Press.
Wagenaar, C. (2020), 'Modern Hospitals and Cultural Heritage' in *Docomomo Journal Special Edition Cure and Care*, no. 62, 2020/01, Lisbon, pp. 36–43.
Wallace, A. (2016), *Ulrike Meinhof's* Bambule: *Performing Politics in the Electronic Public Sphere*, Senior Honors Thesis Department of Germanic and Slavic Languages and Literatures University of North Carolina at Chapel Hill.
Walton, A. (1894), 'The Cult of Asklepios', in *Cornell Studies in Classical Philology*, No. 3, New York: Ginn & Company.

9

Deleuze (and Guattari) and the Concept of Contaminated People

Virgilio A. Rivas

Introduction

'Flight is challenged when it is a useless movement in space, a movement of false liberty' (Deleuze and Guattari 1986, 13). Deleuze and Guattari wrote these lines in a section called 'An Exaggerated Oedipus', challenging the notion of Oedipal conflict as the productive principle behind the construction of neurosis. In their book on Kafka, Oedipus becomes instead a product of desire, which is '*already submissive and searching to communicate its own submission*' (10, emph. in orig.). There is a specific type of coding involved in this so-called 'side communication', thereby creating 'a singular phenomenon' called 'surplus value of code' (Deleuze and Guattari 1987, 53), particularly in light of COVID-19.

Amid the ramifications of this surplus code in a rapidly shifting immunological landscape, what is left of humanity (otherwise, a poor imitation of the ape-code) yielded to a new but autochthonous desire, already tied to the ambivalence of submission. It desires others' submission, just as it is in submission to the signature triangulation of the conflicts of Oedipus. Not just inside the households, but also in schools, factories, assembly lines, etc., dominated by 'bureaucracy as desire ... as an exercise of assemblage itself' (Deleuze and Guattari 1986, 56). In the early months of the pandemic, which, incidentally, the CIA has long predicted (Snowden 2019), the home has exceedingly replaced these spectrums of bureaucracy, this desire for ambivalence, reminiscent of an actual poison: 'poison is only poison by virtue of the fact that the organism directs its activity against it, strives to assimilate it' (Schelling 2004, 56).

When the only correct approach to fight the pandemic was to wait for the contamination curve to flatten no less, the site of the ambivalence of this assimilation occupied the centre stage of the organism's becoming-virus, becoming-plaque. Inside the home, the virus, however, cannot wholly become man itself, just as 'from subsequent impossibilities' it also 'mutates and changes form', such as, in the case of Samsa, from a luckless salesman to a giant insect: Gregor, the literary epitome of a shoddy form of becoming, a 'botched deterritorialization of becomings-animal of [story]' unable to form an assemblage (Stahl 2016, 222). Today, this animal story could not be mistaken for something else. What is the pandemic other than this messed-up becoming-failure of assimilation?

It is a failure so far to the extent that there is no 'maximum of difference or degree of intensity' (Deleuze and Guattari 1986, 22) yet achieved in becoming. On the one hand, since the onset of the pandemic, man's becoming-animal story shows itself capable of a new form of individuation, albeit hooked to visual images and algorithmic feedback and feed-forward loops. At the same time, the virus rages on, requiring quarantine and lockdown protocols (another animal story), morphing the home into one folded bureaucracy, an assemblage in one, absorbing the workplace and the public space. The household becomes a functional home, marked by a particular degree of intensity caused by hybridizing work and new forms of individuation. Altogether, this reinforces a more complex state of *dividuation* within a network of feedback loops, thresholds and recursions to avoid as much as possible the unpredictable outcome of human fallibility, while maximizing fallibility for managing the entropic forces of nature. (Needless to say, COVID-19 is a force of entropy.) A kind of Deleuzian ethology (Fox and Alldred, 2021) emerges at these fluid intersections, creating the home-fold as an immanent ontology.

On the other hand, the becoming-animal of man inside the enclosure is undergoing a curious test of becoming, the flight of the stationary, but unprepared to embrace the antinomial resolution. To stay in the cage is to remain as a constant unit of the assemblage. This way, one continuously connects with desire that sustains the maximum of difference, as yet attained, thus, delaying its becoming-incompletion's fading out into oblivion (in case the virus completely assimilates the man-code, reducing the latter to its elemental form, like the ashes of someone 'thrown into the wind', who has become-molecular after 'entering into a becoming-animal' (Deleuze and Guattari 1987, 116). But also into unencodable chaos into which species life plunges without thinking (expressed no less in the final explosive jubilation of entropy). Here, the Deleuzo-Guattarian Kafka questions the ground of the iterability of liberty as the freedom to assimilate a social code: '("freedom was not what I wanted. Only a way out; right, or left, or in any direction")' (13).

Lastly, amid the alternating refractions of immunology traversing the human and non-human divide, how to achieve that 'maximum of difference' approaches the question of the *refrain*. This concerns the question of which becoming can yield a sort of power capable of creating a new assemblage, 'a new plane of surplus values' (Hammond 2021, 233), which redirects desire away from that logic of submission, the desire to communicate its triangulation into an endless recursive ontology.

The becomings-animal story

The metastable home

At the height of the worst pandemic in human history since the influenza virus, the home has transformed into an intensive object of governmentality, threatening to overdetermine the conventional organological boundary, at least in accepted juridical maxims, between private and public life, autonomy and sociability. The home became akin to paralysis in terms of the impossibility of a line of flight without reproducing or imitating the escape code.

Today, however, some countries have managed the pandemic and are re-opening, or rather, re-enchanting the planes of organic life shut down by a surplus code with calibrated human flows that once characterized a regime of consistency. We are talking about a safe operating space within a pre-planetary dispensation (the pandemic finalizes, as it were, the regime of the planetary) responsible for indexing the madness of fluidity to human flourishing. In turn, this puts the home back to its taken-for-granted autonomy – an enfolded fold, one of the 'two floors of subjectivity' (Deleuze 2006) in the manner of Deleuze's rendition of the Leibnizian monad – which could rejuvenate the desire for in-and-out flights and breakaways from incomplete recursions or delays, which, ironically expressed, defined the optimal index of pre-contamination existence, the *joie de vivre* of the immanence of the pre-pandemic. In a passage from *The Fold: Leibniz and the Baroque*, Deleuze (2006) implies that this taken-for-granted point of inflection, a place such as the home, accommodates autonomous reflection just as much as the experience of delirium like the 'monad's spontaneity [resembling] that of the agitated sleepers who twist and turn on their mattresses' (98). Deleuze writes in one of his reflections:

> For example, I hesitate between staying home and working or going out to a nightclub: these are not two separable 'objects,' but two orientations, each of which carries a sum of possible or even hallucinatory perceptions (not only of drinking, but the noise and smoke of the bar; not only of working, but the hum of the word processor and the surrounding silence . . .) (79).

With the re-enchantment of these indefinite deferrals, life once again offered itself to surplus abstraction.

In hindsight, the absence of intensive regularity of motion that is supposed to amplify the concentration of machinic capture transformed every other rhizome into a digital yet tangible constituent of a technical pre-formatted assemblage, reminiscent of the Kantian manifold. Except here, the Kantian manifold has evolved into a full-blown machinic assemblage, equipped with technical aprioris, all the more predisposed to the necessity of binding existence to the home-fold, in line with the algorithmic management (Berns and Rouvroy 2013) of public health and safety protocols. Algorithms have never been as intense as they were in the most obvious times of stasis.

Here, however, we cannot reduce the disappointment of the rhizome as, for instance, of Gregor Samsa's stationary flight, to the mere expressionism of the individual unit of the home-fold. The rhizome is not independent of the machinic ecology upon which desire imposes an 'image of thought' or a visible spectrum of representation. The assemblage also re-constitutes and re-formulates re-iterable gaps, resumptive flows, fractal interruptions allowing for contingent affirmations of life, *à la* Nietzsche's immanent form of coding within aggregations and networks of flows. The undecided flows within an assemblage may themselves still enable an existing desire for bureaucracy, speaking of human ecologies, on the one hand, and a transempirical, inhuman organology of drives, on the other hand, referring to machines of capture. At any rate, the disappointment reveals an anomalous flow in the assemblage, which reveals itself in terms of '*a posteriori outlining of paths of escape*' (Deleuze and Guattari 1986, 14, emph. in orig.).

In Simondonian terms, this anomaly can be seen from the perspective of the pre-individual milieu, the orthogonal field of impersonal tensions, a metastable horizon offering new lineaments of becomings that are provisional and contingent, but also potentially recursive. As Simondon writes: 'Becoming is in effect perpetuated and renewed resolution . . . proceeding via crises, and as such its sense is in its center, not at its origin or end' (Simondon in Scott 2014, 6). The individual rhizome that expresses this anomaly (what Simondon would call the 'psychic individual') is defined by the relations of tensions that the preindividual milieu generates, which, in turn, gives way to the actual instantiation of the psychic individual within the collective. As Elizabeth Grosz points out, the individual itself unpacks a sort of 'social and collective resonance involving a kind of return to what has been left behind, a retrieval of the remainder' (Grosz 2017, 199). In light of SARS-CoV-2, the 'retrieval' of the metastable can be likened to the return to the household, now the home-fold with social and collective traces concerning the interoperability of individuation techniques against the background of the preindividual.

The result of this interoperability yields a strange tableau of initial conditions for a possible new assemblage, which has since gained a material-semiotic currency, the *new normal*. The pandemic equips this so-called retrieval with a kind of phase shift that enacts a supervening principle. Beyond the twentieth-century model of the separation of the home and the workplace, the pandemic escalates the emergence of an assemblage that complements the twenty-first-century push to connectivity, completely superseding the 'Fordist city' model of the divide between private and public space, which replaced the centralized workstations of the 'industrialized cottage' of the nineteenth century (Doling and Arundel 2020). Throughout these economic shifts, it is not incidental that technology plays a transductive role, in itself a form of 'refusal', echoing Yuk Hui (2015), 'to be reduced to a linear historical process' through its permanent presence in the 'propagation of a structure . . . by passing from one state of energy to another' (Voss 2018). Thus, the divide between private and public space reflects the 'transduction of intensive states' that 'connectivity' as an order of magnitude establishes within a given milieu or space of productivity, thereby '[eventually replacing] topology' (Deleuze and Guattari 1987, 17).

The technological template for such a shift had already been implemented long before the pandemic. The post-Fordist economic shift to 'intangible assets . . . ideas, information, and software' (Doling and Arundel 2020, 4), which line up 'connectivity' with a dominant productive principle, has already 'enabled an expansion of home working to an increasingly wider swath of the workforce' (3). Despite the pervasiveness of the technological capture in pre-pandemic times, however, I argue here that the conditions and apparatuses of capture relative to this specific conjuncture of productivity were still preoccupied with expanding an inception flow, in varying intensities and modulations, to a new obsession with coding. The pandemic paves the way for creating a new machinic phylum within the trajectory of inhuman progress exacerbated by the socio-pathological conditions of societies of control, which Deleuze outlined in his later work, in the guise of 'algorithmic catastrophe'. Yuk Hui (2015) defines this catastrophe as 'the latest development of reason, totally detached from the thinking brain, and becoming more and more significant in our everyday life due to the recent rapid development in artificial intelligence' (125). This inhuman catastrophe is complemented by the ecological ramifications, in light of present climate risks, of multispecies life facing apocalyptic futures, anticipating full-scale inhuman organology that is pure coding.

In 'Postscript on the Societies of Control' (1992), written at the time of the earlybeginnings of globalization, Deleuze specified a metastable state that allows for the 'co-existence' of 'one and the same modulation' (5), predicated on the still overlapping productivity schemes of the past century and the present via the emergence of a 'universal system of deformation' (5). This prompted Deleuze to pursue imaginative futures while problematizing their transductive routes out of the modular flow or passage from one animal to the other, for instance, from the mole to the serpent:

> The old monetary mole is the animal of the spaces of enclosure, but the serpent that of the societies of control. We have passed from one animal to the other, from the mole to the serpent, in the system under which we live, but also in our manner of living and in our relations with others. The disciplinary man was a discontinuous producer of energy, but the man of control is undulatory, in orbit, in a continuous network. Everywhere *surfing* has already replaced the older *sports* (5–6).

Since the modular shift from disciplinary society, the becoming-animal story becomes all the more pronounced as a lexical representation of the inner and external workings of the man-code. Whereas the former society underlined *enclosure*, evocative of the separation of private and public, the society of control paves the way for *modulation* in the manner of 'a self-deforming cast that will continuously change from one moment to the other, or like a sieve whose mesh will transmute from point to point' (4). The becoming-animal story, grasped in terms of networks and energy flows, which we have re-assigned to the changing function of the home vis-à-vis the workplace, comes at a time when the sense of the outside as a limit or threat has already been exhausted; when the 'social field', for instance, 'no longer refers to an external limit that restricts it from above . . . but to immanent internal limits that constantly shift by extending the system, and that re-constitute themselves through displacement' (Deleuze and Guattari 1994, 97). In the larger background of this formulation is the saturation of colonial and imperialist power that had successfully extended its geo-ontological scope to as far as the 'ends of the earth before passing into the galaxy: even the skies became horizontal' (ibid.). A geo-ontological power has since then become completely deterritorialized to the farthest extent of the planet, which inversely corresponds to an 'intension' by capitalism, as Guattari argues, this time '[to infiltrate] the most unconscious subjective strata' (2000, 50). The planetary specificity of this modulation cannot be ignored. The unconscious is the final frontier of the planetary saturation of power. Power is reconstituted via displacement and technological plasticity that serves as the last bastion of territorial modulations whose primary focus is human sensibility or human autonomy (Zuboff 2019). Today, this corresponds to the overdetermination of the so-called 'faciality machine' in terms of modulating the assemblage's new becoming-animal story through the 'social production of the face . . . the facialization of the entire body, and all its surroundings and objects, and the landscapification of all worlds and milieus' (Deleuze and Guattari 1987, 181). Yet this story is not always about the unchallenged linearity of power.

Deleuze and Guattari gave us a prognosis of the extent of restrictions on mobility, which, in a sense, also anticipated the ensuing captivation of the productivity principle by the plasticity of the faciality machine while stuck in a line of stationary escape as humanity chases herd immunity. Notice how the following passages resonate with the experience of being caught in an enclosure in light of periodic lockdowns imposing restrictions upon autonomic flows:

> Even a use-object may come to be facialized: you might say that a house, utensil, or object, an article of clothing, etc., is *watching me*, not because it resembles a face, but because it is taken up in the white wall/black hole process, because it connects to the abstract machine of facialization (175; emph. in orig.).

Incidentally, a 2020 report by the British Council (Darko and Hashi 2020) at the height of the pandemic may offer a partial example of how to challenge the plasticity of the machine of faciality, rebounding as from inhibited fluxes concerning personal and collective autonomy. In short, lockdowns give us an example of outlining a path of escape, despite the odds of not becoming a part of the organism where even minute details cannot elude the white wall's line of sight (the anathema of Gregor Samsa). Where two-thirds of social enterprises (whose respondents span three continents) have diversified their businesses via the massive shift to online platforms, the modulation of use-objects as a body without organs (as opposed to organs without body) is in full play. This is a trend not seen before the worldwide pandemic. This time consumer goods and commodities, echoing a Deleuzian flight of intensity, become 'animated by various intensive movements [determining] the nature and emplacement of the organs' (in this case, the commodity goods and service flows provided by SMEs (small- to medium-sized enterprises) but inhibited by the surplus code of microbial threat disrupting storage, distribution systems and exchange), and that, to a relatively successful degree, have made themselves, these use-objects as an organism in its own right (Deleuze and Guattari 1987, 171–172). As Deleuze and Guattari argue: '[Organs] have to keep enough of the organism for it to reform each dawn . . . to keep small supplies of significance and subjectification, if only to turn them against their own systems when the circumstances demand it' (160). Here the combined modularity of the home-fold and faciality yields a new metastable horizon, though with minimal effect compared with the global economy that integrates parts-objects in the manner of designing a Frankenstein, otherwise an omniscient capital that, like God, 'cannot bear the BwO . . . rips it apart so He can be first' (159). This modularity is an example of absolute coding utilizing less abstract machines for consumption prediction and capture.

The faciality machine

The 2020 pandemic, nonetheless, proved this facialization to be more advanced and, many times over, more effective than the modular resistances to the general economy of social power. Equipped with algorithms supervising over widescale facial action coding system that has remarkably improved since 1978, the once significant interpersonal, even biblical, register of the face exposed to communicative and feedback environments was superseded by an insistent form of coding reducing the face, without dispensing with it entirely, to a re-iterable technical capture. With the face mask, for instance, non-verbal communication is deprived of its naked human connection. The face is supposed to be axially relational, speaking of the 'integration of part-objects' (Deleuze and Guattari 1987, 171) in which affectivity, emotions and feelings, granular details on facial grids involving eyes, mouth, nose and cheeks, play distinct roles. This could bring us back to the scriptures, the 'Ecclesiastes' that Aquinas quoted in *Summa Theologica*: 'The attire of the body and the laughter of the teeth and the gait of the man show what he is' (19, 27). Nonetheless, in terms of the facialization of the body-head, this human face is still a mere signpost of an animal code borne of a 'necessity that does not apply to "human beings"' (Deleuze and Guattari 1987, 170). The facialization of the pandemic exacerbates this body-head's inhuman transmutation into what Deleuze and Guattari describe, in a related criticism of Sartre and Lacan's 'error of appealing to a form of subjectivity', as eyes lacking in gaze, '*gazeless eyes*' or the '*black hole of infinity*' (171). The following recent study on wearing face masks during the pandemic provides a partial context:

> The eyes and the mouth are the two main organs that help in reading others' faces. By wearing face masks, people are inclined to focus more on the eyes to be able to understand the facial expressions intended. Eye contact can be used to show empathy and concern for others, to manage feelings, to express interest, or to help with communication. Nevertheless, prolonged eye contact can result in uncomfortable feelings sometimes, as it can magnify actual interest in communicated material or convey signs of aggression (Mheidly et al. 2020, 2).

The face mask does not escape the faciality machine; on the contrary, it expedites a process of inhuman re/territorialization in the form of imitating an escape code, that of escaping the face to 'become clandestine' (Deleuze and Guattari 1987, 191), which merely doubles the existing animality code. The next becoming-animal story will thus be the success story of another recursive immanent coding whose objective is all-too-familiar, to preempt the rebirth of animality by the anthropogenic capture of the animal code. Notwithstanding its ambivalent opposition to facialization, however, not wanting to become animal can become a codable input to the success story of the inhuman via the faciality's re-doubled 'shining black holes, its emptiness, and boredom' (171). Not wanting to become animal may also turn out to be a serialized enunciation of the animal code.

A recent study related to the pandemic, in terms of the 'perception', not the physical actuality, of the direct gaze, complements this reterritorialization of the white wall in the form of expecting to be seen by an invisible gaze, for instance, in video call interactions during the stay at home policy. (This refers to the expectation of subjective recognition that incidentally TikTok has transformed into an instant global craze.) The study is an addition to the literature on the psycho-physiological response to direct eye contact that the pandemic complicates (Hietanen et al. 2020). This time it is the perception of being seen, not the physical presence of another, that elicits an autonomic nervous response, like smiling or frowning. Other instances further complicate the gaze: '[W]hen the other person was presented just on video, seeing direct gaze elicited the subtle facial reactions of smiling. This suggests that these facial reactions are highly automated responses to eye contact' (University of Tampere 2020).

Arguably, this example can also induct an opening of the face into the realm of 'real multiplicity or diagram with a trait of an unknown landscape, a trait of painting or music' (Deleuze and Guattari 1987, 190); in short, a new assemblage beyond the direct gaze of subjectivity and the landscapification of autonomic response system dependent on physical eye contact that ends up on a white wall, the holey infinity. Still, outside the chatroom, the pandemic becomes this new inhuman necessity for the redoubling of the face, with only the eyes, the vision of the face left to facialize a mask, now a redoubled autonomic nerve response code:

> Either the mask assures the head's belonging to the body, its becoming-animal, as was the case in primitive societies. Or, as is the case now, the mask assures the erection, the construction of the face, the facialization of the head and the body: the mask is now the face itself, the abstraction or operation of the face (181).

Before the modular turn to control society, this vision used to facialize the head, which belongs to the animal dimension of the body through the becoming-animal story of the head from the standpoint of a faciality code. We are referring to the classical treatment of algorithms based on rules that programmers designed. In this sense, ancient Christian writers were pretty much classical coders. The universal face of Christ is a code designed to wield the moral submission of humanity whose animality, or the secular content of their supposedly hallowed origin, rationalizes the necessity of theological redemption. Deleuze and Guattari write: '[T]he face represents a far more intense, if slower, deterritorialization. We could say that it is an *absolute* deterritorialization: it is no longer relative because it removes the head from the stratum of the organism, human or animal, and connects it to other strata, such as signifiance and subjectification' (172).

The success story of faciality in the past did not stop with Christianity. It would be followed by the Renaissance's obsession with portrait painting, then modernity's fascination with photography that has led to the statistical massification of the face into today's cloud storage systems containing data banks via sophisticated machine-learning algorithms.

Meanwhile, so far as it is leading us in other directions, it pays to note that outside China's example with its relatively successful Health Code (Liu 2021), Greece, the birthplace of Western philosophy, was the first to utilize machine algorithms to curb the spread of COVID-19. Nicknamed Eva, this AI is a sophisticated 'reinforcement learning system' with more efficient predictive capability in dealing with 'population-level epidemiological metrics' that random physical testing could not perform (Bastani et al. 2021). The results were impressive, helping Greece to neutralize the effects of the pandemic. But the actual success story of Eva depends on peoples, body-heads facialized into dividuals as 'data banks' (Deleuze 1992, 5) through their mobile phones and smart gadgets, which have become 'woven into [human] routines and produce habituated embodied interaction' (Edensor 2011, 198).

This is the perfect correlate of the facialization of the mask of the body-head where the mask becomes Deleuzian (read: capitalism also behaves like its opponents in a schizophrenic way [Portanova 2015, 96)] terms the sense of 'the production of a continuum of intensities in a nonparallel and asymmetrical evolution' [Deleuze and Guattari 1986, 13]). Stiegler recently expanded this concept (building on Leroi-Gourhan's anthropological works) to mean the 'co-evolution of psychosomatic organs, artificial organs, and social organizations' (2020a, 82). The body-head is not only facialized but intensively masked, revealing the fundamental question of the 'criteria' or the 'occultation' of the 'criteria of *retention*' (2020b, 103). What is being masked and obscured is the metaphysics of the pre-selection of the criteria of becoming-animal story (the retentional element of the story of becoming-animal of man) with the help of the most sophisticated machine-learning algorithms that supersede history, experience and memory.

However, the new necessity for faciality redoubling in light of SARS-CoV-2 is not entirely flawless. We can find in Nietzsche, for instance, an exemplary model of coding as a form of nomadic thought associated with a type of people with a unique approach to uncoding, 'not in the sense of relative uncoding [or] the decoding of codes past, present, and future, but an absolute encoding – to get something through which is not encodable, to mix up all the codes' (Deleuze 2004, 254). The case of commercial algorithms utilized by giant corporations such as Google and Amazon to predict consumer trends deserves a closer look. At the height of the pandemic, historical data became unreliable as vector points to influence the oscillating gradients of consumer behaviour via feedback loops (Wetsman 2020) through as browsing history and digital footprints, traces and inflection points of 'archival metaphysics' (Hui 2018). The crux of the matter is machine-learning algorithms are not like humans who can amuse themselves with causation. These algorithms do not understand the intoxication of humans with meanings affecting their behaviour (Pearl and Mackenzie 2018, 28). Meanings are complex forms of expressiveness derived from 'pure sensory qualities', making their construction closer to art just as much as 'art begins with the animal' in the sense of the animal '[carving] out a territory and [constructing] a house (both are correlative, or even one and the same, in what is called a habitat' (Deleuze and Guattari 1994, 183). But this habitat is also prone to accidents borne of the human propensity for both causation and cause-faulting, producing a peculiar relation between 'endosomatic' (biological or vital) and 'exosomatic' (artificial) forms of co-implicating causalities. Daniel Ross (2021) offers a summary of this point, taking up Deleuze's and Stiegler's philosophical lenses correlative to the pandemic:

> 'Accidentality' is as fundamental to exosomatic différance as it is to vital différance, and exosomatic accidents, too, may often breed monsters but can also prove

> fortuitous – provided that we have the capacity to adopt them, to *make* selections, not biologically but economically and noetically, that is, rationally (in a very broad sense), and thereby to make these accidents into our necessity, our quasi-causal necessity, in Deleuze's terms.

This partly echoes the theory of assimilation that Schelling proposed in the eighteenth century concerning the peculiar nature of the poison. It is not the poison that assaults the body but the reverse. The body seizes the poison (Schelling 2004, 56). Let's say the poison is the correlative of the virus. The outcome of the assimilation of the two is something external to their relation, SARS-CoV-2, the virus that has mutated into another exosomatic fold. One of them is COVID-19, the disease that has originated a quasi-causality entrapped in body natures via an emergent mash-up of pathogens between humans and non-humans.

There is more to this correlation than we have established so far concerning the assimilation of the virus in the body, but let us assume that a social mechanism is masking the disease through the hybridity of the new normal. As a serialization of the overcoding of the disease, the new normal assimilates the virus by striving against it. As we have lost count of the deaths in the process, however, the system creates a 'stationary zone of representation', which is the statistical face of the disease, vis-à-vis a 'mutant flow . . . [eluding] or [escaping] the codes' (Deleuze and Guattari 1987, 219). This brings us to the possibility of contaminated people with a new becoming-animal story to modulate and complicate the persistent code of SARS-CoV-2 by de-subjectifying the anthropogenic vision of ending the pandemic.

Contaminated people

In a short essay by Leonard Lawlor, 'Following the Rats: Becoming-animal in Deleuze and Guattari' (2008), the concept of losing track of death may insinuate itself into the very logic of this new normal in terms of how affects are re-channelled into impersonal statistical aggregates. In this sense, the awareness of death as a passage from one affect to another is masked by the dispassionate autonomy of numerical data. But in the case of 'becoming-rat', Lawlor takes advantage of the modularity of affects that can override the masking of death; to put death instead under the category of zero, to become indiscernible like zero. Death is less a question of termination than of serialization of a refrain (more on this in the concluding section).

Lawlor builds on *A Thousand Plateaus*' discussion of Hugo von Hofmannsthal's fiction 'The Lord Chandos Letter', which gives us an archetype of writing for a people to come through a segmental exchange of affects; people contaminated enough to become capable of exchanging surplus codes with rodents. We are here looking at the tenth Plateau where Chandos, who, let us imagine, was writing back to Francis Bacon, told the latter about his transformation as a writer after witnessing 'the death throes of the pack of rats' (179) that he deliberately poisoned. Chandos was so transformed by the agony of the rats that he decided to write like a rodent. Not out of pity for them but because something remained in the aftermath of trading surplus codes. To clarify, it is not the sinister motive to bring these animals to their deaths that brings out the intensive nature of the transfer, but rather the remainder of the exchange itself.

To use these deaths as leverage (against animal ethics) to evoke an exchange of affects from which a people to come emerges is nothing less than vulgar literalism. In the same vein, as far as science is concerned, COVID-19 is not some premeditated bio-weapon unleashed on the population by a rogue nation-state. But nor is the virus a translator in terms of swapping and switching of codes that produce a controllable outcome. Instead, the virus' side-communicative flow engenders something that defies genealogy, i.e. an *antimemory* (Deleuze and Guattari 1987, 294) that 'takes on a new kind of power' (225). This is the equivalent of 243 million active cases and close to 5 million and counting (non-reterritorializable) deaths worldwide. This is not to mention six variants of the disease while the two latest variants are being monitored by global health authorities, all with unpredictable transmissibility significance and impact.

Nonetheless, the idea of deliberate poisoning may also reflect a modular exercise of the will upon non-human ecologies and habitats responsible for the extinction of lower species, vertebrate species, in particular, that would otherwise take thousands of years to disappear within a natural cycle (Ceballos et al. 2015). Mass extinction has never been as severe as a crisis of multispecies security. Not until humanity's most recent desire for a new becoming-animal story reveals a traumatized psychonoetic life, too prone to the machinic displacement of post-disciplinary society, via the deepening infiltration of the unconscious realm (per Guattari's description). In control society, desire sustains a delirious co-existence of contradictory affects, say, between violence and pity.

As Deleuze and Guattari widely argue, 'desire desires its own repression' (1987, 215), but also its intensive reduction to elemental forms, down to the most fundamental a-signifying, a-subjective level of material composition when desire plunges into chaos, invades ecologies, poisons animals, destroys biodiversity, at the same time being able to witness the handiwork of its violence through apocalyptic futures within an expanding wasteland of dystopian capitulation to dark enlightenment, post-truth and ecological dead ends. These by-now active futures give rise to unpredictable pathogens in a virosphere disrupted by frantic human commerce that upsets multispecies ecologies.

Viruses do not suffer trauma, but diseases are way different. The inherent double bind that makes diseases unfold in bodily natures theoretically makes them suffer traumas as well. But also, bodies and diseases do not outlast each other unless a state of equilibrium intervenes. In post-infection life, a body-disease begins to spawn a different type of body that becomes itself a segment of the planet's germinal life, as before is also already contaminated with elements of non-life, the non-autopoietic workings of bodies without organs, viruses that decimate organisms (Colebrook 2014). Through this post-infection life, the Kafkaesque possibility of a new people emerges, the opposite of a people phenomenologically wired to encounter and immerse in 'lived experiences, Oedipal subjects of conjugal contracts' (Stahl 2016, 231) prone to habitual perversions of thought. Or, the opposite of a people who had known their lives as organs without bodies, known only the sadness that decreases their capability to act just as much as they ignored or were unaware of the intricacies of bodies and how they prompt the passage of affects. Here, the Kafkaesque becoming-animal story conjoins with the

Spinozist body creating a 'micro-physics of affect-constellations' (5), paving the way to a necessary inflection point parallel to the macro-realism of an internalized saturation of social power based on the immanent limits of autonomic flows.

Incidentally, the latter standpoint, a macro-cosmic framework of thinking, acting and intervening, lacks the torsion of an inflection point that corresponds to the new immanence of the centripetal acceleration of fluxes (in the wake of desire's transition to undulatory movement) where displacement and contraction take over the function of expansion and projection. The globalist framework must overwhelm this inflection point as much as its function, besides impeding lines of flight, is to guarantee that the bigger picture of things, a dogmatic image of thought-world, accurately represents a modular re-assignation of the world (already saturated by the planetary) from the outside to the inside (Guattari's domain of the unconscious). The 'bigger picture' is supposed to reflect the fact that there is no more outside, which communicates a new desire for life, so we are told since the beginnings of globalization: 'If where we are is a *globe*, then it can be imagined as delimited, bounded, organically self-referring and unified' (Colebrook 2014, 62). It is in this sense that any notion of people in it, in a literal globalized world will always be a 'disturbing outcome of systemic events' (168), people as an epiphenomenon of systems, assuming that the global centripetal movement of desire is a unilateral failure, which has been going on for decades, especially in light of the pandemic as when warning signs were ignored before the outbreak of COVID-19.

Still, a form of minor literature or becoming-animal story can infract this cycle of desire not to recover the subjective origination of flows but rather to exacerbate it. This comes at a time when the horizontal reduction of the skies that Deleuze and Guattari talked about creates the condition for double immanence when the outside enfolds inward, thus relatively making the inside the new plane of immanence, but also re-creating the intrinsic and extrinsic vectors of molar and modular fluxes within:

> This is where one thinks no longer with figures but with concepts .... There is no longer projection in a figure but connection in the concept. This is why the concept itself abandons all reference so as to retain only the conjugations and connections that constitute its consistency. The concept's only rule is internal or external neighborhood. Its internal neighborhood or consistency is secured by the connection of its components in zones of indiscernibility; its external neighborhood or exoconsistency is secured by the bridges thrown from one concept to another when the components of one of them are saturated (1994, 90).

To the same extent as the concept's inflection from a redoubled plane, a 'correlate of creation' (108) arises alongside creating a new earth, a new plane of consistency. But, as Deleuze and Guattari warned, this correlate, a people to come, will not emerge in existing democracies, in the machinic phylum of body-heads entrapped in faciality. A new plateau of pessimism and despair is food, even oil, for an even more heightened escalation of post-truth. Or a new plane of consistency showing signs of early vexation from having been confined to the planetary grids of optimal human flourishing long enough to want to land on different celestial germinal atmospheres – the absurdly wealthy taking on the prospects of space tourism, Mars colony and beyond. The pandemic aggravates the modular irritation of the capable rich to save the planet from 'sickness unto death', the despair over the pathogenic acceleration of entropy in the face of the irreversibility of climate risks. In short, the rich need their own people, a people they could summon, which is the opposite of those who can gracefully avoid the 'majority' (108).

At the same time, however, COVID-19 has produced shadows of these people to come; people as concept-movements/machines flowing/surfing on 'flat surfaces, without levels, orderings without hierarchy'; thus, in the same manner as one asks 'what to put in a concept' (90), the question of what to place in the neighborhood of a people that is not yet actual, overwhelms the bigger picture of the planet saturated by a false attempt at purity. (The latter drove Heidegger to pursue a people under the banner of the Third Reich.) Just as people are defined by their neighbourhood, so is a concept, by surfaces, levels, plateaus. But until then it is still conceptual, in the process of becoming what it is, such as 'mass-people, world-people, brain-people, chaos people' (218). As with the notion of the future, a people to come can simply 'disappear when they are realized' (218) since their present becoming 'is what [they] are, thereby, what already [they] are ceasing to be' (112).

In a complementing way, COVID-19 has awakened a 'people' from a post-planetary future about to reframe the duration and intensity of a phase shift in terms of thermodynamic relation to entropy. This geological turn will anticipate either a people ready to push back the acceleration of present entropy the sooner they disappear or create the conditions for a post-tellurian world hundreds of years from now (where they would have already disappeared).

Conclusion: a people's refrain

In passing, it pays to note that Derrida, in *The Animal That Therefore I Am* (2008), conveys a proximate vision of a new becoming-animal story vis-à-vis a Kafkaesque animality conjoining with Spinozist body *sub specie aeternitatis*. Derrida instigated quite a similar problematic by expanding the fundamental question, initiated by Bentham, of the possibility of animal suffering. Neither Deleuze nor Derrida assumed that animals do not suffer. Except here, Derrida's vision lacks the specificity of the field of intensive forces that animal becoming through suffering manifests from a Deleuzian perspective. When suffering becomes abominable, grief or anguish 'forewarn' of the 'advent of a people' (Deleuze and Guattari 1994, 110). The becoming-animal enters the becoming-molecular. This is not something that Derrida anticipates. Notwithstanding, there is nothing to prohibit us from inflecting his concept of animal violence to that point of intensive molecularity lacking in his recourse to friendship and justice.

Derrida, for instance, identifies the logic of animal violence 'in the most morally neutral sense of the term' as the logic of masking its cruelty in the name of the 'human animal'. The correlation of non-human suffering and genetic violence has been well established, as Derrida argues, through

> the industrialization of what can be called the production for consumption of animal meat, artificial insemination on a massive scale, more and more audacious manipulations of the genome, the reduction of the animal not only to production and overactive reproduction (hormones, genetic crossbreeding, cloning, etc.) of meat for consumption ... and all of that in the service of a certain being and the putative human well-being of man (2008, 25).

In light of SARS-CoV-2, the Derridean question of the animal may thus highlight the impact of anthropogenic violence leading to a pathogenic, not to mention ecological, crisis. But what do we become after infection? After a severe climate meltdown? In a lengthy passage that follows, Lawlor suggests the writing of tales, becoming-animal tales, for sure, which presupposes a people, not only as consumers of tales but also as their proximal creators and created as well:

> Is this collectivity a people (as in Deleuze) or a democracy (as in Derrida)? .... Perhaps this collectivity to come would be themselves a people who thought feverishly. Haunted by the specter of the agony of animals that they find within themselves, perhaps they would say 'This land that I seem to possess is not my own.' They would say, 'Let's open all the doors and destroy the walls.' Perhaps they would be a people who loved the world so much that they would want to let everyone, without exception, enter in, and to let everyone, without exception, exit out. Perhaps, we could call this people to come 'the friends of passage' (2008, 184).

But 'friendship' is too Derridean, too animal to become a man-code. What friendship lacks is the 'molecular, becoming zero' (Deleuze and Guattari 1994, 169) of a zone of inflection between the animal and man (like 'claimant or rival, but who could tell them apart?' [4]), such that their relation engenders a force or affect wrested from any reference, animal or man, rival or claimant. This force/affect is certainly not a Derridean gift of the moment that may indicate mutuality or hospitality; certainly, not a democracy. Rather, it is a concept, which presupposes co-adaptation. Every concept already belongs, like it or lump it, to 'families of concepts' (77) wrested from their former becoming-animal stories that have become molecular. Every concept is a potential persona, an 'agent of enunciation' (65); not a personal figure, but rather elemental or spiritual, call it demonic, such as one wrestling with *pulsion*, the maximum of difference between drives and symptoms (1983, 23), as if for the first time; a newborn animal that is not yet deterritorialized, one that awaits a new earth.

In democracies, friendship instead gives way to its contradictory complement, such as the travails of Gregor Samsa, who did not lack friends, in the first place. In the social triangulation of Oedipus, friendship is encrusted in the 'machine of judgment and condemnation' (Deleuze and Guattari 1986, 11). All the lines of segmentation are distributed in this triangulation: 'the lines of family and friends, of all those who speak, explain, and psychoanalyze, assigning rights and wrongs, of the whole binary machine of the Couple, united or divided, in rigid segmentarity' (1987, 206). With Facebook transforming into Metaverse, all these will pave the way for a second life of recursive segmentarity; a virtual space as augmented abstract machines, holograms of judgement, but also repeatable praise, accolade, recognition, etc., which are the lineaments of a 'divisible, homogenous space striated in all directions' (223). Perhaps, the proper tailender to Latour's dress rehearsal in the aftermath of the pandemic (to borrow the halting problem theory) is the beginning of the end of the self-iteration of a system: 'We do not lack communication. On the contrary, we have too much of it' (108). Rather, the system has met an executable goal or a proof state in preparing the animal code to enable a new form of contingency. In the context of the pandemic, which we have already assigned to the becoming-animal code, the proof state is that democracies do not work in times of extreme emergency. The proof state is that desire continually desires its own repression, which is the desire for democracy: 'Democracies are majorities' (1994, 108).

Beyond the proof state, democracy has not yet met a contaminated people. But, like a refrain, this concept-movement recurs in an autochthonous form, the autochthon becoming-stranger to herself. The movement recurs in the present, in a territorial assemblage that is territoriality only as far as it allows a passage or other ways of feeling and existing (Wiame 2021, 141). A people to come speak the same language but do not understand themselves; a people 'strangely deformed in [the] mirror of the future' (Deleuze and Guattari 1994, 110); too contaminated, too feverish to stay in one assemblage that no sooner than they reached a house, a territory, 'launch [themselves] on a mad vector as on a witch's broom' (185). Perhaps, to celebrate catastrophe that 'no longer frightens many people' (Chatelet 2000, 9), this new animal bears witness to the 'earth's [passage] into a plane of immanence' (Deleuze and Guattari 1994, 88), a new plane of immanence, and absorbs the earth, assimilates it, like a body does to weed out a poison. In conclusion, these viral people are now the poison that will settle the problem of assimilation by inventing a new organism to complicate, even exaggerate, for creativity to tear down the walls of segmentation, the Body without Organs.

References

Bastani, H., Drakopoulos, K., Gupta, V., Vlachogiannis, I., Hadjichristodoulou, C., Lagiou, P., Magiorkinis, G., Paraskevis, D., and Tsiodras, S. (2021), 'Efficient and Targeted Covid-19 Border Testing through Reinforcement Learning', *Nature*. https://doi.org/10.1038/s41586-021-04014-z.

Berns, T. and Rouvroy, A. (2013), 'Algorithmic Governmentality and Prospects of Emancipation', translated by E. Libbrecht, *Réseaux* 177: 163–196. https://doi.org/10.3917/res.177.0163.

Ceballos, G., Ehrlich, P., Barnosky, A., Garcia, A., Pringle, R., and Palmer, T. (2015), 'Accelerated Modern Human-Induced Species Losses: Entering the Sixth Mass Extinction', *Science Advances 1* (5): e1400253.

Chatelet, G. (2000), *Figuring Space: Philosophy, Mathematics, and Physics*, Dordrecht/Boston/London: Kluwer Academic Publishers.

Colebrook, C. (2014), *Death of the Posthuman, Vol. 1: Essays on Extinction*, New York: Open Humanities Press.

Darko, E. and Hashi, F. M. (2020), *Innovation and Resilience: A global snapshot of social enterprise response to Covid-19*, British Council. https://www.britishcouncil.org/sites/default/files/socialenterprise_covidresponsesurvey_web_final_0.pdf.

Deleuze, G. (1992), 'Postscript on the Societies of Control', *October* 59: 3–7. http://www.jstor.org/stable/778828.

Deleuze, G. (2004), 'Nomadic Thought', in *Desert Islands and Other Texts, 1953–1974*, edited by David Lapoujade and Michael Taomina, 252–261, New York: Semiotex(e).

Deleuze, G. (2006), *The Fold: Leibniz and the Baroque*, translated by Tom Conley, New York: Continuum.

Deleuze, G. and Guattari, F. (1983), *Anti-Oedipus: Capitalism and Schizophrenia*, vol. 1, trans. R. Hurley, M. Seem, and H. R. Lane, Minneapolis and London: University of Minnesota Press.

Deleuze, G. and Guattari, F. (1986), *Kafka: Toward A Minor Literature*, translated by Dana Polan, Minneapolis and London: University of Minnesota Press.

Deleuze, G. and Guattari, F. (1987), *A Thousand Plateaus: Capitalism and Schizophrenia*, translated by Brian Massumi, Minneapolis and London: University of Minnesota Press.

Deleuze, G. and Guattari, F. (1994), *What is Philosophy?* translated by Hugh Tomlinson and Graham Burchell, New York: Columbia University Press.

Derrida, J. (2008), *The Animal That Therefore I Am*. New York: Fordham University Press.

Doling, J. and Arundel, R. (2020), 'The Home as Workplace: A Challenge for Housing Research', *Housing, Theory, and Society*. https://doi.org/10.1080/14036096.2020.1846611.

Edensor, T. (2011), 'Commuter: Mobility, Rhythm, and Commuting', in *Geographies of Mobility: Practices, Spaces, Subjects*, edited by Tim Cresswell and Peter Merriman, 189–203, Farnham, UK: Ashgate.

Fox, N. J. and Alldred, P. (2021), 'Doing New Materialist Data Analysis: A Spinozo-Deleuzian Ethological Toolkit', *International Journal of Social Research Methodology*, https://doi.org/10.1080/13645579.2021.1933070

Grosz, E. (2017), *The Incorporeal: Ontology, Ethics, and the Limits of Materialism*, New York: Columbia University Press.

Guattari, F. (2000), *The Three Ecologies*, translated by Ian Pindar and Paul Sutton, New Jersey: Athlone Press.

Hammond, M. (2021), 'Capacity or Plasticity: So Just What is a Body?', in *Deleuze and the Fold: A Critical Reader*, edited by Sjoerd van Tuinen and Niamh McDonnell, 225–242. New York: Palgrave Macmillan.

Hietanen, J., Peltola, M. J. and Hietanen, J. (2020), 'Psychophysiological Responses to Eye Contact in a Live Interaction and in Video Call', *Psychophysiological*, *57*(6): e13587. https://doi.org/10.1111/psyp.13587.

Hui, Y. (2015), 'Algorithmic Catastrophe – The Revenge of Contingency', *Parrhesia* 23, 122–143.

Hui, Y. (2018), *Archives of the Future. Remarks on the Concept of Tertiary Protention*, Landsarkivet i Göteborg.

Hui, Y. (2021), 'On the Persistence of the Non-modern', *Afterall*, 51, https://www.afterall.org/article/on-the-persistence-of-the-non-modern.

Lawlor, L. (2008), 'Following the Rats: Becoming-animal in Deleuze and Guattari', *Substance* 117 (37/3): 169–187.

Liu, C. (2021), 'Seeing Like a State, Enacting Like Algorithm: Reassembling Contact Tracing and Risk Assessment during the Covid-10', *Science, Technology and Human Values*, https://doi.org/10.1177%2F01622439211021916.

Mheidly, N., Fares, M., Zalzale H., and Fares, J. (2020), 'Effect of Face Mask in Interpersonal Communication During the Covid-19 Pandemic', *Frontier Public Health*, 8: 582191. doi: 10.3389/fpubh.2020.582191.

Pearl, J. and Mackenzie, D. (2018), *The Book of Why: The New Science of Cause and Effect*, New York: Basic Books.

Portanova, S. (2015), 'The Genus and the Algorithm: Reflections on the New Aesthetic as a Computer's Vision', in *Post-digital Aesthetics: Art, Computation, and Design*, edited by David Berry and Michael Dieter, 96–108, New York: Palgrave Macmillan.

Ross, D. (2021), 'The Pandemic Should Not Have Happened', *Melbourne School of Continental Philosophy*. https://mscp.org.au/plague-proportions.

Schelling, F. W. J. (2004), *First Outline of a System of the Philosophy of Nature*, translated by Keith R. Peterson, New York: State University of New York Press, Albany.

Scott, D. (2014), *Gilbert Simondon's Psychic and Collective Individuation: A Critical Guide*, Edinburgh: Edinburgh University Press.

Snowden, F. M. (2019), *Epidemics and Society: From the Black Death to the Present*, New Haven and London: Yale University Press.

Stahl, O. (2016), 'Kafka and Deleuze/Guattari: Towards a Creative Critical Writing Practice', *Theory, Culture & Society*, 33 (7–8): 221–235.

Stiegler, B. (2020a), 'Elements for a General Organology', *Derrida Today*, 13 (1): 72–94.

Stiegler, B. (2020b), *Nanjing Lectures: 2016–2019*, translated by Daniel Ross, London: Open Humanities Press.

University of Tampere (2020), 'Eye Contact Activates the Autonomic Nervous System Even During Video Calls', *ScienceDaily*. www.sciencedaily.com/releases/2020/04/200423130442.htm.

Voss, D. (2018), 'Simondon on the Notion of the Problem: A Genetic Schema of Individuation', *Angelaki: The Journal of Theoretical Humanities*, 23 (2): 94–112.

Wetsman, N. (2020), 'The Algorithms Big Companies Use to Manage Their Supply Chains Don't Work During Pandemics: The Data Algorithms Use Isn't Reliable', *The Verge*, 27 April, https://www.theverge.com/2020/4/27/21238229/algorithms-supply-chain-model-pandemic-disruption-amazon-walmart

Wiame, A. (2021), 'The Refrain and the Territory of the Posthuman', in *Performance and Posthumanism: Staging Prototypes of Composite Bodies*, edited by Christel Stalpaert and Kristof van Baarle, 137–152, Switzerland: Palgrave Macmillan.

Zuboff, S. (2019), *The Age of Surveillance Capitalism: The Fight for a Human Future at the New Frontier of Power*, New York: Public Affairs.

10

On the Difference between Morality and Ethics in the New Normal: Gilles Deleuze's Spinozist Ethics in the Context of COVID-19

Kyle J. Novak

Introduction

The COVID-19 pandemic is often discussed as a single ongoing event. However, there is a distinction we can draw between the physical impersonal appearance of the SARS-CoV-2 virus in the world along with the accompanying COVID-19 disease and human ethico-political response to the disease. The emergence of COVID-19 in the world as a novel disease was met by a host of non-pharmaceutical interventions (NPIs) such as mask mandates and lockdowns as well as new sets of norms around physical distancing all intended to reduce the spread of the SARS-CoV-2 virus. The combinations of NPIs and the norms surrounding it are often referred to as the New Normal and as such we can distinguish it from the COVID-19 pandemic. Much as we can distinguish between the disease COVID-19 and the New Normal, on a Deleuzian account we can distinguish between ethics as a typology of immanent modes of existence (or ethology) and morality as a set of valuations concerned with passing judgement on the ground of transcendent values.

In this chapter I develop an account of Gilles Deleuze's ethics through his work on Spinoza, which he contrasts with morality, to argue that an ethical response to the COVID-19 pandemic should resist the moralizing of the New Normal and instead have an immanent focus on what is happening to us. In the first part of the chapter I detail the novel approach to ethics as ethology that Deleuze works out most explicitly in *Spinoza: Practical Philosophy*. In the second part I show exactly how Deleuze contrasts ethics from morality and moral thinking before showing the relation of ethics to morality in relation to the New Normal and contrast the Deleuzian ethical perspective from other ethical philosophical accounts that I claim are indicative of a moral approach to the New Normal. I conclude by arguing that the prevalence of the New Normal amidst the COVID-19 represents a triumph of what Spinoza calls the sad passions and suggest Deleuze's ethics might be a way to reject those sad passions.

Deleuze's Spinozist ethics

In *Spinoza: Practical Philosophy* (*SPP*), Deleuze reminds us that centuries before Nietzsche's warnings against the nihilistic tendencies of Modernity, Baruch Spinoza had denounced 'all the falsifications of life, all the values in the name of which we disparage life'. For Deleuze, Spinoza's philosophy is in the first place an ethics oriented around the *joy* of living a life characterized by freedom and opposed to the 'sad passions' or values that disparage life, including: sadness itself, hatred, fear, aversion, anger, indignation, despair, cruelty and even security.[1]

Spinoza's admonition against the sad passions comes from his theory of the affects in the *Ethics* (*E*) where he argues that those affects which contribute to joy lead us toward perfection while those that involve sadness lead us away from perfection.[2] For Spinoza, to be more or less perfect means to be more or less real (*E*III, General Definition of the Affects) and a thing is more or less real insofar as it is better able to 'persevere in its being' or exist as whatever kind of thing that it is (*E*IIIP6). When it comes to humans, our ability to persevere in our being (i.e. survive) is correlated to the power of our body to act and the power of our mind to think (*E*IIIP11). Thus, anything which contributes to joy is necessarily good for us while anything that contributes to sadness is necessarily bad.

On Deleuze's reading then, Spinoza's ethics requires a denunciation of the sad passions because life is an impossibility if we are overcome by those passions: 'We do not live, we only lead a semblance of life; we can only think of how to keep from dying, and our whole life is a death worship' (*SPP*, 26). The life of sad passions spent concentrating on death is not so much a matter of an individual's ethical shortcoming as it is a matter of the political workings of a society. The proliferation and persistence of the sad passions comes from what Deleuze calls 'the moralist trinity' of the slave, the tyrant and the priest. The slaves are those who possess sad passions which are exploited by the tyrant and facilitated by the priest 'so that they will fight for their servitude as if they were fighting for their own deliverance'.[3] That is, a despotic state is one that uses its power to mobilize the sad passions – fear, hatred, etc. – so that citizens will make themselves slaves by trading their freedom for a sense of safety. In contrast, a 'true city' is one that 'offers citizens the love of freedom' (*SPP*, 26).

For Deleuze, the tendency of societies to move toward tyranny and the sad passions rather than freedom and joy was the question that motivated Spinoza in his political writings: Why are people 'proud of their own enslavement? Why do they fight "for" their bondage as if it were their freedom?' Underlying all of these, Spinoza wonders: 'Why are the people so deeply irrational?' (*SPP*, 9–10). Yet, if we pause here for a moment to turn these questions back on Spinoza/Deleuze, we can uncover a tension in the framework that Deleuze provides: Are the people really irrational? Are security and freedom, in fact, antithetical? If, on the contrary, it is the case that security is sometimes needed to guarantee safety, which is a pre-condition for the possibility of any freedom; then it would only be rational to occasionally embrace the sad passions and trade some freedom for security.

That trade is, of course, the locus of the social contract which stands at the foundation of the tradition of Western political philosophy beginning with Hobbes and running throughout liberal theory. Spinoza himself will appeal to both the state of nature and need for a social contract when he observes that 'there is no one who does not wish to live in security and so far as that is possible without fear; but this is very unlikely to be the case so long as everyone is allowed to do whatever they want and reason is assigned no more right than hatred and anger' (*TPT*, 197). How is it then that Spinoza can claim that a desire for security is universal if such desiring invokes the sad passions? I will address that in due course. However, to do so I first want to highlight how the tension does not just exist at the level of politics and affects but goes to the heart of Deleuze's understanding of Spinoza's ethico-ontology.

Spinoza's monistic philosophy operates through what Deleuze refers to as the doctrine of parallelism. That is, in contrast to Descartes' ontology where reality consists of the two substances, mind (*res cogitans*) and body (*res extensa*), Spinoza posits that all of nature is comprised of a single substance that expresses both the attribute of thought and the attribute of extension. The two attributes do not interact yet in every way that a body expresses itself there is a corresponding or parallel expression in thought. Therefore, to say that an affect contributing to joy empowers us or that an affect of sadness disempowers us means that both the body's power to act and the mind's power to think are effected. In other words, joy and sadness for Spinoza do not just describe psychological or mental states as any expression of the mind is accompanied by a corresponding expression of the body.

The doctrine of parallelism shows that there are two possible ways in which we can be subject to the sad passions. In the first place, we can see why Deleuze thinks that a life controlled by the sad passions is only a semblance of living. A mind that is subject to the sad passions is not one that is free because fear, anger, etc. usurp the mind's power to think. And, according to the doctrine of parallelism, if the mind's power to think has been diminished by sadness then the body's power to act must also be diminished. We might call this sort of subjection to the sad passions a *constraint through affect*. Instances of this sort of constraint become apparent in the context of the New Normal. From fear of the SARS-CoV-2 virus or legal repercussions, many people did not leave their houses or refused to partake in social gatherings in a sort of self-imposed house arrest or solitary confinement. In other instances it may not have been fear of the virus itself that constrained people. It has been commonplace for people to avoid friends or family out of fear of the guilt they might experience if an infection followed a gathering. Similarly, many people avoided socializing or forms of recreation they used to enjoy for fear of the shame they might suffer if anyone were to witness them not behaving according to the norms of the New Normal.[4] In all these cases, the body is not constrained from acting due to physical restraint but is nonetheless literally constrained by the affects.

In contrast to constraint through affect, we may think of those cases where the body is physically restrained as *constraint through motion*. Here we get to the heart of Deleuze's understanding of Spinoza's ethico-ontology that I mentioned above. Up to this point I have emphasized the affective dimension of Spinoza's ethics but just as there is a parallel between mind and body there is another parallel that Deleuze conceptualizes in terms of two axes: '*longitude* and *latitude*' (*SPP*, 127). The latitude is the set of affects pertaining to a given thing while longitude refers to the sets of relations involving the movement – speed and slowness, motion and rest – of any given thing. Mind and body, longitude and latitude, affect and motion: Deleuze will say that Spinoza's ethics is constituted through these various complementary sets which are ways of adequately expressing things through parallelism. He calls Spinoza's approach to ethics an ethology which is not only an ethics but also an epistemology whereby we can understand things in terms of what they do and an ontology where what a things does can be expressed through both a dynamic (affective) and kinetic (motion) proposition (*SPP*, 123). I won't give a more detailed account of ethology here as that is something I explore elsewhere.[5] To explain this, a bit must be said about what I mean by constraint through motion.

At various points in *SPP*, Deleuze explains that in addition to affect, we can understand things through 'compositions of relations' (*SPP*, 12, 58, 126). Spinoza's ontology posits that there are elemental or 'simple' bodies that form relations with one another and thereby come to compose more and more complex bodies where the whole of Nature can be conceptualized as a complex body of which every other body is a part (*E*IIL1-*E*IIL7N). To say that any-thing causes or undergoes a change is to say that its composition of relations has changed, which is to say that some or all of its parts have *moved* in such a way that their relationship has been altered. Despite the talk of simple/complex bodies we should not forget that parallelism means that to speak of an alteration of the body is to speak of an alteration of the mind. Deleuze describes the whole process in the following way:

> When a body 'encounters' another body, or an idea another idea, it happens that the two relations sometimes combine to form a more powerful whole, and sometimes one decomposes the other, destroying the cohesion of its parts. And this is what is prodigious in the body and the mind alike, these sets of living parts that enter into composition with and decompose one another according to complex laws. The order of causes is therefore an order of composition and decomposition of relations, which infinitely affects all of nature. But as conscious beings, we never apprehend anything but the *effects* of these compositions and decompositions: we experience *joy* when a body encounters ours and enters into composition with it, and *sadness* when, on the contrary, a body or an idea threaten our own coherence (*SPP*, 19).

This ethological framework that Deleuze provides allows us to account for anything whatsoever in terms of compositions of relations changing through motions. To give a very basic example, the processes of attaining nourishment by eating food are an instance of our body encountering another and entering into a composition with it. We could describe this relationship in any of three ways that amount to the same thing: the nourishment leads our power to increase, we move toward perfection by better persevering in our being, and we experience joy. To give another example related to the New Normal: the disease COVID-19 is determined by the presence of the SARS-CoV-2 virus in a human body. That is, COVID-19 refers to the composition of relations between virus and host. In the worst cases the relation formed between virus and host is one which leads to the decomposition of the host to the point where the host no longer persists in its being (i.e. cases where the outcome is death).

What I have called constraint through affect and constraint through movement both amount to the same thing – albeit expressed in different ways – that is, some subjection to a sad passion which leads to a decrease in power/capacity to act/freedom. For example, a person who is unable to leave their house because they are afraid of contracting COVID-19 or afraid of the consequences of violating a stay-at-home order is just as unfree as the person who is unable to leave their house because their ability to move has been compromised by COVID-19. In Deleuze's ethico-ontological terms, we might say that both cases are bad for the person concerned in that some sadness (due to a constraint through affect in the former cases and constraint through movement in the latter) has produced a decrease in their power or capacity to act. Herein I think lies a clarifying point on the tension between security and safety and freedom. On this account, limiting what one can do in the name of security is necessarily to give up some freedom. Such limitations necessarily involve the sad passions in that giving up freedom means a decrease in joy accompanying the decrease in one's power to act. Likewise, if a freely made action leads to some decrease in one's power to act (i.e. a harm), then the sad passions are involved as well. That is to say – on Deleuze's account of Spinoza – there are some situations that necessarily involve the sad passions. To say that a thing experienced no sad passions would be to say that the thing only experiences joy, which would be to say that the thing is perfect, which is only applicable to God or the whole of nature and not finite entities (modes) such as humans.

The framework that Deleuze develops through his reading of Spinoza can – I think – clarify the tension that we saw earlier. Ultimately, there are no situations where we possess perfect freedom, which in Spinoza's terms means that our joy is always somewhat tempered by sadness. Therefore, something that might appear to be security isn't really a compromise with the sad passions insofar as it has a net positive on our capacity to act. The challenge for reason is to be able to discern between those situations where security (in one sense) leads to an increase in freedom and those where security (in a second sense) is in fact a compromise with the sad passions that unnecessarily limits our capacities for action. For the sake of clarity, I'll use the word *safety* to refer to matters in the former sense and reserve *security* for cases of the latter. Thus we can slightly modify Spinoza's claim above from *TPT* to read 'there is no one who does not wish to live in safety and so far as that is possible without fear'. And recalling the next part of the claim, we can say that safety is promoted when our action is curtailed (either by our own volition or an external force) in accordance with reason. In contrast, through security constraints in the name of safety are done out of fear or anger or hatred and ultimately decrease our powers of action. The only ethical dilemma we face if we accept the Deleuzian Spinozistic meta-ethical framework (ethology) is whether some course of thinking or action will ultimately lead to an increase or decrease of our capacities for action.

In some ways the COVID-19 pandemic has been the test case *par excellence* for such a dilemma. On the one hand, there is the New Normal which uses a litany of NPIs that limit movement and use surveillance in an effort to reduce viral spread and thereby mitigate the harms the virus could cause. In ethological terms we could say that the *raison d'être* of the New Normal is to do whatever is necessary to create that composition of relations wherein all extant SARS-CoV-2 viruses in existing relationships with human hosts are least able to form new relations with (i.e. infect) other potential human hosts. The SARS-CoV-2 virus can only persist in its being when it is in relation with a human host, so COVID-19 exists as a viral–human assemblage. As such, actions taken in order to prevent the formation of compositions of relations between humans and SARS-CoV-2 (i.e. new cases) are not directed at the virus itself, but at any human body which is potentially a host of the virus. Although the presence of symptoms has traditionally been the marker of disease, COVID-19 is well known for its asymptomatic cases – instances where a human–viral assemblage exists but without any perceivable alteration of relations beyond what a diagnostic test can reveal.[6] The existence of asymptomatic cases means that all human bodies are potential hosts at all times and as such the New Normal conceives of the human as primarily a disease vector. In order to achieve its goal, then, the New Normal operates through the imposition of limitations on the capacities of human actions which could potentially bring any human body into proximity (i.e. '6 feet') with any other human body. In practical terms these impositions have taken the form of border closures, workplace closures, school closures, prohibitions on public gatherings, prohibitions on private gathering, prohibitions on sexual activity between adults from different households (in the UK), stay-at-home mandates, mandates on the wearing of 'non-medical' masks in public places, and mandates requiring proof of vaccination to participate in public life. From an ethological standpoint, the impositions of the New Normal would be rational if they improved safety such that the limitations placed on our powers to act by the impositions were less than the limitations on our powers to act that would result from a greater incidence of COVID-19 resulting from the absence of those impositions. However, the New Normal would be irrational if the constraints resulting from the New Normal itself were greater than the constraints that would be caused by a greater incidence of COVID-19 in absence of the impositions of the New Normal.

Ethics against morality in Deleuze

Looking at things through the lens of ethology – especially something as complicated as the New Normal – is no doubt complex and complicated and it may even seem as futile as attempting a sort of utilitarian calculus that weighs the utils of one course of action against another. Despite the complexity, for Deleuze, it is at least not impossible because it uses life on a shared plane of immanence as a standard. In *A Thousand Plateaus* (*ATP*) he and Guattari use the terminology of ethology to explain this explicitly:

> In any case, there is a pure plane of immanence, univocality, composition, upon which everything is given, upon which unformed elements and materials dance that are distinguished from one another only by their speed and that enter into this or that individuated assemblage depending on their connections, their relations of movement. A fixed plane of life upon which everything stirs, slows down or accelerates. A single abstract Animal for all the assemblages that effectuate it.[7]

We all live in the same physical reality and can witness the alterations that things – living or otherwise – undergo, and the changes that they can affect. In practical terms this means that the world we live in is one that we can perceive and know, and understanding is not a sacred domain reserved for the priestly class of experts. In other words, ethics as ethology is concerned with whatever is actually happening and insofar as we want to understand life we ought to understand what is happening. In *The Logic of Sense* (*LS*), Deleuze says that this goes to the heart of ethics itself: 'Either ethics makes no sense at all, or this is what it means and has nothing else to say: not to be unworthy of what happens to us.'[8] Deleuze understands being worthy of what happens to us in terms of Nietzsche's *Amor fati* – the love of fate. To love fate is not to be resigned to or ignorant or indifferent of what is happening, but rather to be able to confront what is happening without resorting to moralizing or succumbing to the sad passions. Returning to *SPP*, Deleuze will say that a difference between ethics and morality is that the latter is overly concerned with procuring judgement rather than understanding what is happening so 'all that one needs in order to moralize is to fail to understand' (*SPP*, 23). Why is it that morality which is concerned with judgement is characterized by misunderstanding?

Deleuze further defines ethics as he understands it in relation to Spinoza through a contrast with morality by explaining that: 'Ethics, which is to say, a typology of immanent modes of existence, replaces Morality, which always refers existence to transcendent values. Morality is the judgment of God, the *system of Judgment*. But Ethics overthrows the system of judgement. The opposition of values (Good-Evil) is supplanted by the qualitative difference of modes of existence (good-bad)' (*SPP*, 23). To say that ethics is a typology of immanent modes of existence is to say that it operates according to the ethological framework I delineated above. Following Nietzsche again, what we are concerned with when we think about things ethically is not with making the proper judgement – or having 'the right take' – about some matter deemed to be Good or Evil. Rather, ethics is concerned with how bodies are affected and moved in such ways that they enter into compositions of relations whereby their powers are strengthened or diminished. In contrast, morality demands that we pass judgement in accordance with transcendent values which necessarily distracts us from what is actually happening in our immanent reality. And when we replace knowledge of immanence with the command of transcendent moral law, we take ourselves to be either Gods or sinners and cannot help but err as: 'the command is mistaken for something to be understood, obedience for knowledge itself' (*SPP*, 24).

We can see the distinction between ethics and morality in terms of the contrast I made earlier between safety and security. In the case of safety we learn about ourselves and our environments and act in such a way that our capacities for action are promoted as best as possible. In contrast, security demands that we relinquish our abilities to act in the name of some good, but unlike safety which involves learning and knowledge, our action here is motivated by ignorance where knowledge is replaced by an appeal to the moral good. In terms of the New Normal: an ethical approach would require us to understand what is happening and then respond in the way that best mitigates the sad passions. Meanwhile, a moral approach would have us act in accordance with whatever is commanded of us in the name of whatever is judged to be good, regardless of the facts of the situation at hand.

Ethics against morality in the New Normal

Deleuze's portrayal of the moral course of action might seem like a strawman or a caricature of any sincerely held philosophical position. However, there are peer-reviewed publications on COVID-19 and ethics that seem to have taken exactly such a position. In proceeding I will briefly consider a couple of these 'moral' approaches to the New Normal before concluding with an ethical consideration of the New Normal – i.e. a consideration of what is actually happening.

In an article published a few months into the New Normal titled 'COVID-19 Calls for Virtue Ethics', the authors note a tension between the value of freedom and the impositions put in place by the New Normal through lockdowns. For the authors, this tension exists only if we understand freedom in terms of what Isaiah Berlin termed 'negative liberty' or a view of 'freedom as absence of constraints' (by the state) where the aim of freedom is for each individual to maximize their pleasure at the expense of all else.[9] The authors suggest that such a framework is inadequate because: 'A global pandemic is, within living memory, a novel situation that affects everyone without distinction .... The current situation calls everyone, with or without governments restrictions, to act morally in actions and intentions.'[10] Acting morally means cultivating desires in accordance with nebulously defined virtues wherein we will ourselves 'to give up a little in order to gain moral integrity'. Once we have moral integrity our desires will no longer be directed against constraint and instead we will desire to comply with the restrictions or recommendations imposed by the New Normal 'because this is what a *virtuous person does*'.[11] On such an account, morality takes precedence even over life itself, as the authors note that while we do not know the costs of lockdowns, they may still be prudent even if 'it is true that the costs of lockdown measures may be greater (in terms of human lives even) than the benefit'.[12] In other words, then, morality asks us not merely to acquiesce to constraint but to actively embrace the sad passions so that we desire our own constraint even if the outcome of that constraint is itself a further reduction in our power up to and including the loss of life itself.

It's worth taking a moment to consider the two claims that the authors say call us toward morality. In the first place they note that a global pandemic is novel within living memory. This claim is a fine example of moral thinking being used to obfuscate from what is really happening, as other pandemics in the past century are a matter of public record, with influenza pandemics occurring in 1957–1958 (H2N2 Virus), 1968 (H3N2 Virus) and 2009 (H1N1 Virus). But are those pandemics in anyway comparable to COVID-19? Here we should recall the Deleuzian ethical maxim and consider what is actually happening to us rather than leap to moral invocation. In the cases of the 1957–1958 and 1968 pandemics, the U.S. CDC estimated that there were about 1.1 million and 1 million deaths worldwide.[13]The 2009 pandemic was considerably less severe with only about 200,000 deaths.[14] For comparison, just over 1.8 million deaths were directly attributed to COVID-19 in 2020 although the WHO estimated that number could be as high as 3 million.[15] For the comparison to be meaningful we should also keep in mind the growing population of Earth where 1.1 million people in 1957 constituted the same percentage of the human population as would 3.062 million in 2020, and 1 million in 1968 is the same percentage of the population as 2.194 million in 2020.[16] Of course, the disease COVID-19 did not begin and end with 2020, but as a single year event its severity was not novel in living memory. Rather, the first year of COVID-19 was comparable to the influenza pandemics of the second half of the twentieth century. And while those influenza pandemics were single year events, the strains that caused them continue to exist to this day and are counted amongst seasonal influenza strains, claiming a comparably mild 400,000 lives in a given year.[17]

As an ongoing event not limited to 2020, the disease COVID-19 is – at the time of writing – responsible for almost exactly 5 million deaths and we can expect that number to grow as time continues to pass.[18] Accordingly, we would be justified to say that while comparable to pandemics of the second half of the twentieth century, COVID-19 has been responsible for proportionally more deaths and therefore constitutes a novel situation in living memory. However, if living memory does not exclude the oldest living humans, then we should also account for the 1918–1919 H1N1 influenza pandemic. According to the CDC, the 1918 pandemic was responsible for at least 50 million deaths – about an order of magnitude more than COVID-19.[19] Adjusted to the 2020 population, a pandemic of comparable severity today would claim more than 215 million lives. Even worse, the age group most likely to experience fatal outcomes from the 1918 pandemic was 15–34-year-olds in contrast to COVID-19 where those 85 years of age and older are at the highest risk of death and have accounted for the greatest number of deaths, at least in the United States according to data from the CDC.[20, 21] As a result, the 1918 Pandemic was even worse in terms of potential 'life' lost rather than just 'lives' lost.

The point of all this is that while COVID-19 has been and continues to be a disease that has led to millions of deaths, that fact hardly makes it novel. Instead, by the measure of the twentieth and earlier twenty-first century, COVID-19 represents an outbreak of infectious disease more severe than some, comparable to others, and more than an order of magnitude less severe than the H1N1 of 1918. The fact that disease outbreaks comparable to COVID-19 are not novel is not significant for the disease COVID-19 itself (i.e. the disease COVID-19 is exactly as bad insofar as it causes decompositions of relations of human bodies that correspond to decreases in power), but it is significant for thinking about the New Normal. The New Normal calls us to think and act morally in the face of a new and unknown threat. It tells us that new norms are needed if we are to preserve ourselves because the old norms are now unsuitable. Indeed, the New Normal tells us that without the norms of the New Normal, the situation would be unimaginably worse despite the fact that some jurisdictions have refused to implement the norms which studies have shown not to impact mortality.[22] However, from an ethical standpoint untroubled by morality, we can look around at the present reality and recognize it is not so different from the old.

From an ethical standpoint, the edict of the New Normal now becomes open for questioning. Recall that the *raison d'être* of the New Normal is to do whatever is necessary to create that composition of relations wherein all extant SARS-CoV-2 viruses in existing relationships with human hosts are least able to form new relations with (i.e. infect) other potential human hosts. The authors of the call for virtue ethics echo this with the blanket claim that 'it would be bad for human beings to be infected with SARS-COV-2 and to infect others'.[23] Infection with the virus is necessarily bad from a moral standpoint and therefore we ought to avoid infection and avoid any activity (i.e. being in physical proximity with other human bodies as they are disease vectors) which might lead to infection.

Why is infection necessarily bad? One of the possible outcomes of infection with SARS-CoV-2 is an asymptomatic case where the virus is present in a composition of relations with the human body but produces no alterations or constraints to the body itself in terms of either affect or motion. In such cases, infection is – from an ethical standpoint – neither good nor bad. This is definitionally true as there is no alteration to the body and no corresponding alteration (either an increase or decrease) to the body's capacities for action. Of course, there are still some potentially bad outcomes if an asymptomatic infection leads to another infection that is not asymptomatic, but such are not the terms set by the morality of the New Normal. As the aim of the New Normal is to minimize cases – regardless of the outcome of any cases – any case is a bad case. Here we can recall the second claim made by the virtue ethicists as to why COVID-19 calls us to morality: the situation is not just one that is novel, but one that *affects everyone without distinction*.

Some variation of that second claim has been a central tenet of the New Normal both among philosophers and the wider discourse. Writing in *Vox* in the early days of the New Normal, Sarah-Vaughan Brakman, a Professor of Philosophy at Villanova University, argues that the physical distancing demanded by the New Norm is a duty rather than a choice as she repeats the mantra '*We are all in this together*'. The claims that we are affected without distinction and are in this together are meant to elicit a response of solidarity wherein we recognize that 'we face a common threat' while doing 'our part by holding each other accountable, as we hold each other dear (but not too near)'.[24] Almost identical to Brakman's call for an equal-but-separated solidarity, Andrew Benjamin argued in *Philosophy Today* in Fall 2020 for a solidarity stemming from the disconnect between the 'non-discriminatory nature of the virus' and 'settings that are inherently discriminatory' where all bodies are vulnerable to the virus but where outcomes differ due to 'disequilibria of power'. The claim that the virus does not discriminate is taken up by Benjamin who notes that it is a common claim made about SARS-CoV-2 that even appeared in the title of a press release for the United Nation's Office of the High Commission for Human Rights.[25]

The mantras that the virus does not discriminate, that it affects all without distinction, and that we are all really in this together are ostensibly empirical claims but are in fact part of the moral law of the New Normal. As the New Normal is categorically opposed to new cases the avoidance of infection becomes a categorical imperative. To become a positive case is to violate the imperative where on the one hand the non-discriminatory nature of the virus means that any case is as bad as any other. On the other hand, the fact that we are all in this together means that an individual infection is not merely an individual failure but a failure for all, and we must hold each other accountable to avoid such failings. However, from an ethical standpoint, the virus is highly discriminatory. In some cases, entering into a relation with the virus leads to that worst possible outcome (death). Other cases, as I mentioned above, may produce no perceptible alteration of our capacities, no alteration of joy or sadness, no symptoms.

In terms of understanding what is happening to us, understanding the likelihood of different possible outcomes matters. But how do the best case and worst case scenarios stack up? According to a systematic review and meta-analysis of 350 studies on asymptomatic SARS-CoV-2 infection published in the *Proceedings of the National Academy of the Sciences* (PNAS), the likelihood of asymptomatic infection is 35.1 per cent, or just over one in three cases, where younger people are more likely to be asymptomatic.[26] At the opposite end of the spectrum, CDC projections show exactly how discriminatory the virus is in terms of age among individuals without immunity from vaccines or prior infection. For paediatrics, they estimate that exactly 1 death will occur in every 50,000 cases (0.002 per cent of cases). Among those under 50 this rises to 1 death in every 2,000 cases (0.05 per cent), with the majority of these being at the older end of the age range. The outcomes are considerably worse for older adults at 1 in every 166 cases (0.6 per cent) and those over 65 fare the worst by far, with 1 death for every 11 cases (9 per cent).[27]

Concluding thoughts: a triumph of the sad passions?

The picture painted by considering what is actually happening is not one of a radically novel virus or a virus that doesn't discriminate. That picture is radically different than the one painted by the New Normal and yet the triumph of the New Normal in many countries around the globe suggests that the promise of safety is really a mask for security. That is to say, the picture presented according to the New Normal is not reflective of what is actually happening, and is instead indicative of an embrace of the sad passions.

The influence of the sad passions – that is, as Spinoza frames it, evidence of people's desire to work for their bondage as if it were their freedom – is apparent when we consider the relationship between perceptions of the disease COVID-19 with its actual impact. In most cases we find that people have tended to gravely overestimate the risk to their safety from the disease. To give an example of this, the Brookings Institute conducted a survey at the end of 2020 of 35,000 US adults according to party affiliation. Two of their findings stand out. Both Republicans and Democrats dramatically overestimated the likelihood of COVID-19 infection leading to hospitalization. Almost half of Democrats and nearly a third of Republicans estimated that at least 50 per cent of infections lead to a hospitalization. Yet only a quarter of Republicans and fewer than one in ten Democrats correctly estimated the actual number, which is between 1 and 5 per cent, and less than 4 per cent of respondents underestimated that number. Similarly, the perception of who is at risk was much more in line with the New Normal *all in this together* narrative than with the data. Both parties estimated that people over 65 accounted for less than half of deaths, when in reality that age group accounted for more than 80 per cent of deaths. In contrast, people identifying with both parties estimated that around 8 per cent of deaths were in people 24 and younger, when in reality that cohort only accounted for 0.1 per cent of deaths.[28, 29]

The evidence suggests that the demands of the New Normal do not become a rational assessment of risk in terms of what is actually happening to us, but from the influence of sad passions such as fear and anger. Yet the real indicator of the sad passions is revealed by considering the one thing the New Normal seems to disregard – that is, every decrease in our capacities stemming from the New Normal not resulting from COVID-19. I won't detail these but will close by quickly noting two. In the United States alone, working people saw their wealth and the relative power that comes through economic security decrease by $1.3 trillion dollars as a result of the New Normal.[30] Meanwhile, billionaires consolidated their wealth by 54 per cent or almost $4 trillion between March of 2020 and March 2021.[31] Globally, the picture is far worse and estimates suggest that while over 1 billion people had exited extreme poverty (living on less than $1.90 per day) since 1999, the New Normal pushed between 119 to 124 million people back into extreme poverty.[32] As a final remark, if we consider the sad passions in the more limited yet literal sense of mental well-being, then the devastation of the New Normal is evident. Even though young people stand a less than a 1 in 50,000 chance of dying from COVID-19, they have not been so resilient to the New Normal. In Canada, paediatric hospitals reported more than a 100 per cent increase in admissions for mental health problems while admissions for substance abuse and attempted suicide rose by at least 200 per cent.[33]

Overall, the promise of the New Normal to save lives has, for many – especially the most vulnerable – led to a semblance of life. From a moral standpoint the New Normal blackmails us with a call to follow its decrees or be personally responsible for murder even while doing so has led to a dramatic increase of the sad passions and a loss of capacity for action. But from the alternative standpoint of Deleuze's Spinozist ethics, which cares not for judgement but asks us to be worthy of what is happening to us, we can consider an alternative. The alternative is one that again comes from Deleuze where, after examining what is happening, we might consider the unhappy demands of morality and answer simply: 'I would prefer not to.'

Notes

1 Deleuze, G. (1981) 1988, *Spinoza: Practical Philosophy*, trans. R. Hurley. San Francisco: City Lights Books, 26.

2 Spinoza, B. (1677) 2005, *Ethics*, trans. E. Curley, London: Penguin Classics, EIII, definitions of the affects, II–III. Hereafter referred to parenthetically in the text using a standard notation for Spinoza: Book-Part-Proposition number or Definition, Postulate, Scholium, Lemma etc. where necessary, as represented here.

3 Spinoza, B. (1670) 2007, *Theological-Political Treatise* (*TPT*), trans. J. Israel and M. Silverthorne, Cambridge and New York: Hackett Publishing Company, 6. See also, *SPP*, 25.

4 An entire paper could easily be written on the role of shame and shaming in the New Normal so I won't discuss it in detail here, but one rather spectacular example is illustrative of how strong a role it has played. In March and April of 2020, a Florida

lawyer named Daniel Uhlfelder began dressing up as the Grim Reaper and went viral posting pictures on his Twitter @DWUhlfelderLaw in costume at the beaches to shame other beach goers.

5 Novak, K. (2021), 'We Still Do Not Know What a Body Can Do: The Replacement of Ontology with Ethology in Deleuze's Spinoza', *Symposium* 25 (2): 75–97.

6 'Glossary: Centre for Evidence-Based Medicine (CEBM), University of Oxford' (n.d.), https://www.cebm.ox.ac.uk/resources/ebm-tools/glossary (accessed 30 October 2021).

7 Deleuze, G. and F. Guattari. (1980) 1987, *A Thousand Plateaus: Capitalism and Schizophrenia*, trans. B. Massumi, 2nd edn, Minneapolis: University of Minnesota Press, 255.

8 Deleuze, G. (1969) 1990. *The Logic of Sense*, trans. M. Lester and C. Stivale, New York: Columbia University Press, 149.

9 Bellazzi, F. and K. Boyneburgk (2020), 'Covid-19 Calls for Virtue Ethics', *Journal of Law and Biosciences* 7 (1): 1–8, 2.

10 Ibid., 3.

11 Ibid., 8 (emph. in orig.).

12 Ibid., 6.

13 '1957–1958 Pandemic (H2N2 Virus) | Pandemic Influenza (Flu) | CDC' (2019), Centers for Disease Control and Prevention, https://www.cdc.gov/flu/pandemic-resources/1957-1958-pandemic.html (accessed 30 October 2021). '1968 Pandemic (H3N2 Virus) | Pandemic Influenza (Flu) | CDC', (2019), Centers for Disease Control and Prevention, https://www.cdc.gov/flu/pandemic-resources/1968-pandemic.html (accessed 30 October 2021).

14 '2009 H1N1 Pandemic'. (2019) Centers for Disease Control and Prevention, https://www.cdc.gov/flu/pandemic-resources/2009-h1n1-pandemic.html (accessed 30 October 2021).

15 'The True Death Toll of COVID-19: Estimating Global Excess Mortality' (n.d.) World Health Organization, https://www.who.int/data/stories/the-true-death-toll-of-covid-19-estimating-global-excess-mortality (accessed 31 October 2021).

16 'World Population by Year' (n.d.), Worldometer https://www.worldometers.info/world-population/world-population-by-year/ (accessed 1 November 2021).

17 'The Spanish Flu (1918–20): The Global Impact of the Largest Influenza Pandemic in History' (n.d.), Our World in Data. https://ourworldindata.org/spanish-flu-largest-influenza-pandemic-in-history (accessed 1 November 2021).

18 'Home' (n.d.), Johns Hopkins Coronavirus Resource Center. https://coronavirus.jhu.edu/ (accessed 1 November 2021).

19 '1918 Pandemic (H1N1 Virus) | Pandemic Influenza (Flu) | CDC' (2020), Centers for Disease Control and Prevention, https://www.cdc.gov/flu/pandemic-resources/1918-pandemic-h1n1.html (accessed 1 November 2021).

20 'The Discovery and Reconstruction of the 1918 Pandemic Virus' (2019), Centers for Disease Control and Prevention, https://www.cdc.gov/flu/pandemic-resources/reconstruction-1918-virus.html (accessed 1 November 2021).

21 'COVID-19 Provisional Counts – Weekly Updates by Select Demographic and Geographic Characteristics' (2021), https://www.cdc.gov/nchs/nvss/vsrr/covid_weekly/index.htm (accessed 27 October 2021).

22 For example, one analysis at the country level published by the *Lancet* found that: 'Rapid border closures, full lockdowns, and wide-spread testing were not associated with COVID-19 mortality per million people.' C. Rabail, G. Dranitsaris, T. Mubashir, J. Bartoszko, and S. Riazi (2020), 'A Country Level Analysis Measuring the Impact of

Government Actions, Country Preparedness and Socioeconomic Factors on COVID-19 Mortality and Related Health Outcomes'. *EClinicalMedicine* 25 (August).

23 Bellazzi, F. and K. Boyneburgk (2020), 'Covid-19 Calls for Virtue Ethics', *Journal of Law and Biosciences* 7 (1): 1–8, 2.

24 Brakman, S. (2020), 'Social Distancing Isn't a Personal Choice. It's an Ethical Duty' (2020), Vox, https://www.vox.com/future-perfect/2020/4/9/21213425/coronavirus-covid-19-social-distancing-solidarity-ethics (accessed 31 October 2021).

25 Benjamin, A. (2020), 'Solidarity, Populism and COVID-19: Working Notes', *Philosophy Today* 64 (4): 833–837, 824–825.

26 Pratha, S., M. Fitzpatrick, C. Zimmer, E. Abdollahi, L. Juden-Kelly, S. Moghadas, B. Singer, and A. Galvani (2021), 'Asymptomatic SARS-CoV-2 Infection: A Systematic Review and Meta-Analysis', *Proceedings of the National Academy of Sciences* 118 (34).

27 'Healthcare Workers' (2020), Centers for Disease Control and Prevention. https://www.cdc.gov/coronavirus/2019-ncov/hcp/planning-scenarios.html.

28 Rothwell, J. and S. Desai (2020), 'How Misinformation Is Distorting COVID Policies and Behaviors'. *Brookings* (blog), 22 December 2020. https://www.brookings.edu/research/how-misinformation-is-distorting-covid-policies-and-behaviors/.

29 For a more complete analysis of this topic, see also: Brown, R. (2020), 'Public Health Lessons Learned from Biases in Coronavirus Mortality Overestimation', *Disaster Medicine and Public Health Preparedness* 14 (3): 364–371.

30 Cohen, S. (2020), 'U.S. Workers Have Lost $1.3 Trillion – So Why Is Stimulus on Hold?' Forbes. https://www.forbes.com/sites/sethcohen/2020/05/19/us-workers-have-lost-13-trillion---so-why-is-stimulus-on-hold/ (accessed 2 November 2021).

31 'Billionaires Got 54% Richer during Pandemic, Sparking Calls for "Wealth Tax"' (2021), https://www.cbsnews.com/news/billionaire-wealth-covid-pandemic-12-trillion-jeff-bezos-wealth-tax/ (accessed 2 November 2021).

32 'Updated Estimates of the Impact of COVID-19 on Global Poverty: Looking Back at 2020 and the Outlook for 2021' (2020), https://blogs.worldbank.org/opendata/updated-estimates-impact-covid-19-global-poverty-looking-back-2020-and-outlook-2021 (accessed 2 November 2021).

33 McArthur, B., N. Racine, and S. Madigan (2021), 'Child and Youth Mental Health Problems Have Doubled during COVID-19', *The Conversation*, http://theconversation.com/child-and-youth-mental-health-problems-have-doubled-during-covid-19-162750 (accessed 2 November 2021).

References

'1918 Pandemic (H1N1 Virus) | Pandemic Influenza (Flu) | CDC' (2020), Centers for Disease Control and Prevention, https://www.cdc.gov/flu/pandemic-resources/1918-pandemic-h1n1.html (accessed 1 November 2021).

'1957–1958 Pandemic (H2N2 Virus) | Pandemic Influenza (Flu) | CDC' (2019), Centers for Disease Control and Prevention, https://www.cdc.gov/flu/pandemic-resources/1957-1958-pandemic.html (accessed 30 October 2021).

'1968 Pandemic (H3N2 Virus) | Pandemic Influenza (Flu) | CDC', (2019), Centers for Disease Control and Prevention, https://www.cdc.gov/flu/pandemic-resources/1968-pandemic.html (accessed 30 October 2021).

'2009 H1N1 Pandemic' (2019), Centers for Disease Control and Prevention, https://www.cdc.gov/flu/pandemic-resources/2009-h1n1-pandemic.html (accessed 30 October 2021).

Bellazzi, F. and K. Boyneburgk (2020), 'Covid-19 Calls for Virtue Ethics', *Journal of Law and Biosciences* 7 (1).

Benjamin, A. (2020), 'Solidarity, Populism and COVID-19: Working Notes', *Philosophy Today*, 64 (4): 833–837, 824–825.

'Billionaires Got 54% Richer during Pandemic, Sparking Calls for "Wealth Tax"' (2021), https://www.cbsnews.com/news/billionaire-wealth-covid-pandemic-12-trillion-jeff-bezos-wealth-tax/ (accessed 2 November 2021).

Brakman, S. (2020), 'Social Distancing Isn't a Personal Choice. It's an Ethical Duty' (2020), Vox, https://www.vox.com/future-perfect/2020/4/9/21213425/coronavirus-covid-19-social-distancing-solidarity-ethics (accessed 31 October 2021).

Brown, R. (2020), 'Public Health Lessons Learned From Biases in Coronavirus Mortality Overestimation', *Disaster Medicine and Public Health Preparedness* 14 (3): 364–371.

Cohen, S. (2020), 'U.S. Workers Have Lost $1.3 Trillion – So Why Is Stimulus On Hold?' Forbes. Accessed November 2, 2021. https://www.forbes.com/sites/sethcohen/2020/05/19/us-workers-have-lost-13-trillion---so-why-is-stimulus-on-hold/.

'COVID-19 Provisional Counts – Weekly Updates by Select Demographic and Geographic Characteristics' (2021) https://www.cdc.gov/nchs/nvss/vsrr/covid_weekly/index.htm (accessed 27 October 2021).

Deleuze, G. (1981) 1988, *Spinoza: Practical Philosophy*, trans. R. Hurley. San Francisco: City Lights Books.

Deleuze, G. (1969) 1990. *The Logic of Sense*, trans. M. Lester and C. Stivale, New York: Columbia University Press, 149.

Deleuze, G. and F. Guattari. (1980) 1987, *A Thousand Plateaus: Capitalism and Schizophrenia*, trans. B. Massumi, 2nd edn, Minneapolis: University of Minnesota Press.

'Glossary: Centre for Evidence-Based Medicine (CEBM), University of Oxford' (n.d.), https://www.cebm.ox.ac.uk/resources/ebm-tools/glossary (accessed 30 October 2021).

'Healthcare Workers' (2020) Centers for Disease Control and Prevention. https://www.cdc.gov/coronavirus/2019-ncov/hcp/planning-scenarios.html.

'Home' (n.d.) Johns Hopkins Coronavirus Resource Center. https://coronavirus.jhu.edu/ (accessed 1 November 2021).

J. Rothwell and S. Desai (2020), 'How Misinformation Is Distorting COVID Policies and Behaviors.' *Brookings* (blog), December 22, 2020. https://www.brookings.edu/research/how-misinformation-is-distorting-covid-policies-and-behaviors/.

Novak, K. (2021), 'We Still Do Not Know What a Body Can Do: The Replacement of Ontology with Ethology in Deleuze's Spinoza', *Symposium* 25 (2).

McArthur, B., N. Racine, and S. Madigan (2021), 'Child and Youth Mental Health Problems Have Doubled during COVID-19', *The Conversation*, http://theconversation.com/child-and-youth-mental-health-problems-have-doubled-during-covid-19-162750 (accessed 2 November 2021).

Pratha, S., M. Fitzpatrick, C. Zimmer, E. Abdollahi, L. Juden-Kelly, S. Moghadas, B. Singer, and A. Galvani (2021), 'Asymptomatic SARS-CoV-2 Infection: A Systematic Review and Meta-Analysis', *Proceedings of the National Academy of Sciences* 118 (34).

Rabail, C., G. Dranitsaris, T. Mubashir, J. Bartoszko, and S. Riazi (2020), 'A Country Level Analysis Measuring the Impact of Government Actions, Country Preparedness and Socioeconomic Factors on COVID-19 Mortality and Related Health Outcomes', *EClinicalMedicine* 25 (August).

Spinoza, B. (1670) 2007, *Theological-Political Treatise* (*TPT*), trans. J. Israel and M. Silverthorne, Cambridge and New York: Hackett Publishing Company.

Spinoza, B. (1677) 2005, *Ethics*, trans. E. Curley, London: Penguin Classics.
'The Discovery and Reconstruction of the 1918 Pandemic Virus' (2019), Centers for Disease Control and Prevention, https://www.cdc.gov/flu/pandemic-resources/reconstruction-1918-virus.html (accessed 1 November 2021).
'The Spanish Flu (1918–20): The Global Impact of the Largest Influenza Pandemic in History' (n.d.), Our World in Data. https://ourworldindata.org/spanish-flu-largest-influenza-pandemic-in-history (accessed 1 November 2021).
'The True Death Toll of COVID-19: Estimating Global Excess Mortality' (n.d.), World Health Organization, https://www.who.int/data/stories/the-true-death-toll-of-covid-19-estimating-global-excess-mortality (accessed 31 October 2021).
'Updated Estimates of the Impact of COVID-19 on Global Poverty: Looking Back at 2020 and the Outlook for 2021' (2020), https://blogs.worldbank.org/opendata/updated-estimates-impact-covid-19-global-poverty-looking-back-2020-and-outlook-2021 (accessed 2 November 2021).
'World Population by Year' (n.d.), Worldometer https://www.worldometers.info/world-population/world-population-by-year/ (accessed 1 November 2021).

11

The Ethics of Paranoia: How to Become Worthy of COVID-19

Jernej Markelj

The ethics that Gilles Deleuze and Felix Guattari devise in *Anti-Oedipus* is one of empowerment through transformation. Their ethical aim is 'to schizophrenize' our unconscious inclinations and thus release them from the 'territorialities' (that is, specific objects, aims or arrangements) that they invest. By displacing the limits that circumscribe these territorialities and mark out our own territorial identities, Deleuze and Guattari's schizoanalysis seeks to unburden our unconscious activity and mutate it. The limits in question here are equally a matter of borders that we perceive as constituting our biological bodies, our private property, our nation states and our social positioning (class, race, gender etc.). In *Crowds and Power*, Elias Canetti makes a sweeping categorical claim regarding the limits articulating our social existence. He proposes that '[a]ll the distances which men create round themselves are dictated by [the] fear' of being touched (1981, 15). In his view, this allegedly primordial human fear is the central organizing force of our social stratification. 'All life, so far as he knows it,' claims Canetti, 'is laid out in distances – the house in which he shuts himself and his property, the positions he holds, the rank he desires – all these serve to create distances, to confirm and extend them' (ibid.). Different societies might ground these distances differently, some privileging one's birth, others property or profession, but they are all established to keep people apart and prevent unwanted tactile contact between them.

Whether or not we accept Canetti's claim, there is no doubt that in the time of COVID-19 the fear of being touched has become intensified. The fright of contracting coronavirus has not only made us hyper-aware of physical contact with potentially compromising bodies and objects, but has also sensitized us to coughs and sneezes, which – when heard in public spaces – are perceived as offensive. If we merely sniffle or feel vaguely tired or feverish, this anxious scruple is extended to our own bodies. We fear that our bodies are no longer our own, that their supposed functional unity has been compromised by the virus. Deleuze and Guattari refer to the instinctive inclination to maintain distances and police the limits of any established order of things as *paranoia*. Paranoiac tendencies can seek to protect the limits of a heathy body, shielding them from viroid infections, or the borders of a state, which are safeguarded from foreign intruders. As maintaining the invested order can only be achieved by repression directed toward oneself and others, the aim of schizoanalysis is to transmute paranoia and free it from its associated territorialities.

Deleuze and Guattari maintain that paranoiac investments arise spontaneously as our unconscious inclinations inevitably invest our particular social arrangement, as repressive as it might be. In the case of the COVID-19 pandemic, our fears and anxieties are grounded in the unconscious investments of limits and distances prescribed by the measures aiming to contain the virus and the discourse surrounding them. In addition to compulsory handwashing and masks, these measures include strict travelling constraints, the closure of nonessential businesses, prohibition of public gatherings and social events and, in extreme cases, the round-the-clock self-isolation of individuals in their homes. By investing these highly restrictive measures, our unconscious tendencies come to align themselves with that which confines them, or, to put it in Deleuze and Guattari's terms, to desire their own repression. This atomized existence of COVID-19 is akin to Michel Houellebecq's vision of humanity (2000, 2005, 2011), which, due to the decay of its social bonds and institutions, ends up in a technologically assisted alienation. The era of lockdowns and social distancing can be also seen as an intensified version of Canetti's vision of our social world. To avoid touching, Canetti suggests, a 'man stands by himself on a secure and well-defined spot, his every gesture asserting his right to keep others at a distance. He stands there like a windmill on an enormous plain, moving expressively; and there is nothing between him and the next mill' (1981, 16–17).

According to Canetti, the only way to liberate oneself from the fear of being touched is to be immersed in a crowd which erases all borders and distinctions between bodies. In his view, 'all are equal there; no distinctions count not even that of sex' (1981, 15). Canetti adds that the 'feeling of relief [from the burdens of distance] is most striking where the density of the crowd is greatest' (1981, 16). Deleuze and Guattari, conversely, seek liberation from paranoia by schizophrenizing the tendencies that drive us to police the invested limits, which are the very limits that constrain us. Schizoanalysis is a radical treatment that aims to produce 'a line of flight', which de-organizes our paranoid investments, thus allowing us to break free from the unconscious inclinations that ground our responsibilities (1983, 322). To draw a line of flight means to be no longer invested in maintaining a particular order of affairs, to be unbothered and untouched by its disruption.

But would this actually be desirable in our current scenario? The schizophrenizing of our paranoid investments empowers us as it unshackles our unconscious activity from the limits that restrain it. Instead of being exploited for sustaining the socially imposed hierarchies of power, our vital energies can be consequently invested in a more enabling manner. Yet, shaking off the sense of obligation in relation to the coronavirus safety measures might be a different story. There is no doubt that the COVID-19 security plan easily lends itself to biopolitical manipulation. Our situation, suggests Philipp Sarasin, 'looks like a biopolitical dream: governments, advised by physicians, impose pandemic dictatorship on entire populations' (2020). Indeed, Italian philosopher Giorgio Agamben was quick to point out that epidemiology is just another effort to inflict totalitarian control over every aspect of human life.[1] Still, while health and survival can in fact become a pretext for authoritarian manoeuvres, the scientific reports and statistics would have us believe that the threat of COVID-19 is real. If we have not yet completely lost faith in our destabilized consensus reality, we are thus inclined to think that disobeying the safety measures would pose a serious health risk to ourselves and others. In other words, paranoiac investments in coronavirus restrictions seem to work for our own good.

Since in our situation to schizophrenize paranoia becomes an unworkable ethical injunction, a different approach to ethics is required. My chapter seeks to rethink Deleuzian ethics for the time of intensified paranoia. Drawing on *Anti-Oedipus* (Deleuze and Guattari 1983), I begin by situating the COVID-19 pandemic within the libidinal dynamic of the capitalist social formation. I examine how the capitalist market economy brings about fragmentation, or schizophrenization, of culture, and explain how the pandemic, by interrupting the flows of goods, services and labour force, and imposing a set of strict restrictions and lockdowns, results in a wide-ranging paranoia. Building on this analysis, I suggest that the cultural fragmentation instigated by capitalism, and aided by the rise of networked technologies, is reflected in a new situation in which paranoid tendencies invest increasingly divergent social realities. The vectors of this situation, I suggest, can help us understand what has been referred to as the 'post-truth' condition. Drawing on Deleuze's analysis of Nietzsche's *ressentiment*, an illness that he sees as having highly ambiguous effects, I then start to formulate an ethics of paranoia. Like every other illness, I suggest, paranoia does not only inhibit our capacities to act, but, in doing so, also opens us up to new existential outlooks. Remaining faithful to Deleuze's spirit of affirmation, I speculate on what it means to explore these vistas and thus 'become worthy of what happens to us' under the threat of coronavirus (1990, 155).

Paranoia, COVID-19 and the civilized capitalist machine

To situate the COVID-19 pandemic and the paranoiac responses it incites within our contemporary social situation, we need to first explicate what Deleuze and Guattari see as the libidinal dynamic of 'the civilized capitalist machine' (1983, 222). The two libidinal poles that shape this dynamic turn on the innovative model of the unconscious presented in *Anti-Oedipus* (1983, 340). For Deleuze and Guattari, the unconscious should be primarily understood in terms of production. In particular, they see unconscious desire as a productive force that is the motor of all activity and the agent of historical change. This unconscious production 'is never organized on the basis of a pre-existing need or lack' but is entirely positive (1983, 28). The unconscious understood as a factory has no specific aims or objects; it is a pure process that seeks only its own proliferation. When unrestrained, desiring-production functions indiscriminately with whatever is conductive to its proliferation, and is, as such, a matter of fluidity, indeterminacy and change. It is this unrestricted productive process that Deleuze and Guattari align with schizophrenia.[2]

To maintain a social order, each society has to find ways to straight-jacket this schizoid desiring-production. As suggested by Deleuze in his lectures on *Anti-Oedipus* (1971), a society does not fear famine, need or scarcity, but 'is only afraid of one thing: the deluge' of this unrestrained productive energy. To avoid having its social order dissolved by the potent fluidity of desire, each social formation has to 'see to it that no flow [of desire] exists that is not properly dammed up, channeled, regulated' (Deleuze and Guattari 1983, 33). This regulation is achieved by putting on productive activity a set of limitations, which, by giving rise to paranoid tendencies, guarantee that production occurs in a certain way. The despot, for example, reigns by terror, which demands obedience to his law. He uses a variety of intimidation techniques and displays of violence to channel desiring-production into the domain of required labour and away from rebellion. Straight-jacketing of desire is achieved through enforcing a more or less fixed constellation of 'codes', which are constitutive of beliefs. These beliefs concern limits, distances and duties, which prescribe what should be done *today, tomorrow and forever*.

Deleuze and Guattari claim that capitalism functions in a fundamentally different way from pre-capitalist societies as it is intrinsically disruptive. In their view, capitalism is 'the only social machine that is constructed on the basis of decoded flows, substituting for intrinsic codes an axiomatic of abstract quantities' (1983, 139). Instead of reproducing itself through stable systems of beliefs, capitalism arranges its production through axioms, monetary calculations operating solely with quantities.[3] To realize profit, capital recurrently assembles labourers, machines, raw materials and know-how. Axioms bring together these productive factors based on monetary considerations (such as cost-effectiveness), which rule over all political, religious and moral codes. Axioms, unlike codes, as Jason Read suggests, 'do not require belief in order to function' (2008, 145).[4] As it constantly rearranges society irrespective of coded restrictions, capitalist production presents an ongoing disruption to every established order. Correspondingly, Marx and Engels famously suggest that

> [c]onstant revolutionizing of production, uninterrupted disturbance of all social conditions, everlasting uncertainty and agitation distinguish the bourgeois epoch from all earlier ones. All fixed, fast-frozen relations, with their train of ancient and venerable prejudices and opinions, are swept away, all new-formed ones become antiquated before they can ossify. All that is solid melts into air (1848).

In addition to production, consumption, too, is organized by money and subject to ceaseless revolutionizing as managing of consumer tastes constantly refreshes demand for ever-new products and services.

As capitalist social formation erodes all restrictions (be it that of tradition or of last season's fashion), it unleashes desiring-production so it is free to proliferate and form new unrestrained connections. Yet, not to completely undermine its own foundations, capitalism needs to contain this schizophrenic pole of its libidinal dynamic. Capitalism, claim Deleuze and Guattari, 'produces an awesome schizophrenic accumulation of energy or charge, against which it brings all its vast powers of repression to bear' (1983, 34). This recapturing and co-optation of the unleashed desire is achieved by means of the state institutions, corporate bureaucracies, advertising and other antiquated ideologies, but also the nuclear family, which re-constitute subjects as workers, consumers and law-abiding citizens. Unlike pre-capitalist societies, they suggest, capitalism, 'is incapable of providing a code that will apply to the whole of the social field', but instead operates through fragmented sets of *ad-hoc* beliefs that are ancillary to the operations of axioms (1983, 34).

'Capitalism,' claim Deleuze and Guattari, 'restores all sorts of residual and artificial, imaginary, or symbolic territorialities, thereby attempting, as best it can to recode, to rechannel persons who have been defined in terms of abstract quantities' (ibid.). These fragmented make-shift beliefs, which include everything from folkloric nationalisms to fashion trends, in their view make 'the ideology of capitalism "a motley painting of everything that has ever been believed"' (ibid.). As these apparatuses and their fragmented ideologies distribute responsibilities and impose restrictions on desire, they reinforce paranoiac tendencies, which seek to preserve the invested order of things. For Deleuze and Guattari, all our unconscious investments fall between these two poles of desire: the unrestrained, schizophrenic pole and the repressive paranoid one (1983, 340). Insofar as our subjectivities are stable, they are inevitably grounded in durable investments into a particular order of things and are thus to a certain extent paranoid.

Yet, in the time of COVID-19, this libidinal dynamic of capitalism is profoundly transformed. With the measures to contain the virus put in place, the economic activity organized by axioms comes to an abrupt halt. While it is still difficult to assess its overall impact, there seems to be a general agreement among economists that the pandemic is a global economic shock like no other. As the movement of people becomes restricted, the supply chains are interrupted, and stock markets crash, the disruptive activity of capitalist production is slowed down, or, in some sectors and territories, nearly suspended. Since the economic activity at least momentarily frees desiring-production from the potentially exploitative and oppressive aims that it was assigned, Deleuze and Guattari see this schizoid pole as the positive moment of capitalist dynamics. With the schizophenizing movement of capitalism inhibited, this dynamic lands on the side of paranoia, which is associated with the power that seeks to impose a certain kind of order. This paranoid ordering of the world in the time of pandemic, as noted, corresponds to the restrictions enforced by the COVID-19 safety measures. These qualitative measures lay down distinctions between the allowed and the forbidden, the safe and the unsafe, the healthy and the infected etc.

A motley painting of everything that has ever threatened us

Yet it could be argued that, under the conditions of fragmentation brought about by the escalating spiral of capital, this intensified paranoia plays out differently than in pre-capitalist societies. The despotic (or 'barbaric') social machine, for instance, could persist only by enforcing absolute systems of beliefs, which are permanently applicable to the entire social field. The despot, who is, as shown by Canetti, the supreme figure of paranoia, upholds a single standard of value, one that judges as good only that activity that brings him glory.[5] Yet, I have noted that under capitalism such distinct consensus reality is increasingly eroded by the economic operations of the market. In the absence of a coherent ideology, the meaningless calculus of the market is complemented with fragmented, often archaic, beliefs that are established ad hoc.

This fragmentation is further intensified by technologies developed by capitalist production.[6] In particular, this disintegration of our shared social world can be attributed to the effects of digital networks, which have profoundly disrupted our ways of acting and thinking. While the infinitely complex and far-reaching social effects of digital technologies are yet to be fully grasped, the erosion of the common frame of reference, which I see as the defining feature of what has been referred to as the post-truth condition, is hard to deny. As it has provided channels for a decentralized dissemination of information, Nick Land maintains that 'the epistemological authorities have been blasted apart by the internet' (Bauer and Tomažin 2017). According to him, '[w]hether it's the university system, the media, financial authorities, the publishing industry, all the basic gatekeepers and crediting agencies and systems that have maintained the epistemological hierarchies of the modern world are just coming to pieces at a speed that no one had imagined was possible' (ibid.).

The effects of such a destabilization of consensus reality are gravely felt. Its most prominent manifestation is, of course, the *fake news* phenomenon. The traction that alternative political accounts and smearing campaigns have gained online in recent years indicates an effective displacement of a clear limit between the true and the untrue in relation to an increasing number of political issues. The breaking down of consensus is happening also in relation to what a few years ago seemed like indisputable scientific facts, e.g. the existence of global warming or even the shape of our planet. In addition to that, a similar plurality of views is proliferating in relation to nutrition and vaccination. The spreading resistance to the latter foreshadowed the difficulties with the dissemination of the coronavirus vaccine that many countries are facing.

Under these conditions, it would seem that scepticism is no longer the domain of critical thought (what Paul Ricoeur famously called 'the hermeneutics of suspicion') but is becoming a default epistemological attitude. Yet, these paranoid ways of thinking and knowing (which are not directly caused by paranoid unconscious inclinations, but are nevertheless in affinity with them) are not univocally invested in, for example, identifying the offences against the despot's glory. In opposition to pre-capitalist societies, then, paranoid ways of knowing under capitalism are invested in policing increasingly different kinds of social realities. This plurality is evident also in the response to the COVID-19 outbreak. Unsurprisingly, conspiracy theories, which Jameson sees as 'a poor man's cognitive mapping', spontaneous making sense of, and situating oneself within, a situation way too complex to adequately represent, have been proliferating (1988, 356). According to some, the spread of coronavirus has been caused by 5G mobile phone networks, while others have attributed it to polio vaccines.

In the view of Giorgio Agamben, the misrepresentation and coercion have been in fact coming from the side of governments and international institutions. In a series of articles, Agamben has been insisting that coronavirus is a harmless flu used by the Italian state as a pretext to introduce what he has previously theorized as the state of exception (i.e. the suspension of legal order and extension of state power in the wake of a crisis). 'It is almost as if with terrorism exhausted as a cause for exceptional measures, the invention of an epidemic offered the ideal pretext for scaling them up beyond any limitation,' he suggested (2020) when the number of infected in Italy was peaking. Without going too deep into Agamben's analysis, which also includes fierce condemnation of masks, one might be tempted to speculate that his paranoid intervention aims at maintaining a reality in which the state of exception serves as a universal explanatory concept.

For Benjamin Bratton, the proliferation of conspiratorial paranoia is not unexpected. Acknowledging the pressures of being embedded in all-pervasive networked systems that govern more and more aspects of our social reality, coupled with the omnipresent injunction to act as autonomous subjects, he suggests that it is '[n]o wonder that people think that the 5G cell towers are melting the boundaries of their egos' (2021). In response to the propagation of misinformation and conspiratorial accounts, The World Health Organization (WHO 2020) has stressed the urgency of managing what has been referred to as the *infodemic*, 'an overabundance of information', which 'includes deliberate attempts to disseminate wrong information to undermine the public health response and advance alternative agendas of groups or individuals'. Yet, it is fair to add that intense paranoid responses are not only present with the coronavirus- and vaccine-deniers, but also with the people seeing themselves as 'scientifically minded'. While the former group uses social media to try to 'red-pill' the latter and awaken them from their dogmatic slumber, the second group polices being vaccinated as the sharp boundary that separates the intelligent from the delusional.[7] It is certainly true that most conspiratorial accounts are easy to discredit, but the views of the scientific community with regard to the side-effects of the COVID-19 vaccine are not quite as monolithically unanimous as is often presented. As the benefits of the vaccine are still largely seen to outweigh the possible adverse reactions to it, the existing scientific reservations do not advise against vaccination. Still, they do suggest the above-mentioned boundary is perhaps a bit more porous than is sometimes presented.

The ambiguity of paranoia

We should, I believe, acknowledge that such epistemological disorientation is, and will likely become, increasingly so, a default mode of our social existence. Still, if we are not yet completely distrustful of our social reality and its institutions, I suggest the first step in our consideration of Deleuzian ethics would be to accept that coronavirus presents a genuine threat. There is enough evidence which indicates that this is the case, and while COVID-19 is indeed a flu, research decisively suggests that its mortality rate is more than thirty times higher than with regular influenza. It is more difficult to be certain about the involvement of deliberate efforts in spreading the virus, augmenting its spread, or exploiting it politically. Even if the knowledge of such systematic deception was effectively attainable, Eve Sedgwick indicates that this might not be the preferred starting point for a more affirmative ethical approach to our situation.

In her famous essay on paranoia (Kosofsky Sedgwick 2003), she reflects on an answer given by her friend, an activist scholar, to her question about the involvement of the US military in spreading the 1980s AIDS epidemic. Sedgwick's friend responds that she was never really interested in this, and that knowing that this is in fact the case might not change anything. This leads Sedgwick to consider the alternatives to paranoid suspicion, which has in her view become the affective default for the methodology of twentieth-century critical thought. 'To know that the origin or spread of HIV realistically might have resulted from a state-assisted conspiracy,' Sedgwick claims, is 'separable from the question of whether the energies of a given AIDS activist intellectual or group might best be used in the tracing and exposure of such a possible plot' (2003, 124). To put forward an ethical and epistemological approach that is less inhibiting, but has enabling performative effects, she conceptualizes what she calls 'reparative' reading practices (2003, 146–151).

Deleuzian ethics, conversely, pursues a similar goal, that is, empowerment, but does so from a different starting point. I have noted that, for Deleuze and Guattari, the site of the transformative empowerment is the productive unconscious. Yet, as the schizophrenizing of the limits prescribed by COVID-19 preventative measures, and invested by paranoid tendencies, might prove as destructive to oneself and others, I will, as anticipated, explore different approaches to Deleuzian ethics. In particular, since the paranoid tendencies during the pandemic seem to actually work in our favour, my approach will aim to explore the positive potentials of paranoia. This is admittedly a counterintuitive approach as – even if Deleuze and Guattari in *Anti-Oedipus* admit that a degree of paranoia is necessary for a minimally structured existence – they clearly see it as both the effect and the agent of repression, and, thus, their ethical and political enemy.

Still, my contention is that Deleuze offers other venues to explore ethics, and that his affirmative approach can be productively employed even in the times when intensified paranoia is effectively advantageous. My exploitation of an ethics of paranoia is grounded in the idea of illness presented in Deleuze's account of Nietzsche. In *Nietzsche and Philosophy* (1983), Deleuze puts forward an intricate analysis of *ressentiment*, an affective condition that is in some ways similar to paranoia. He suggests that for Nietzsche *ressentiment* is an illness, and one that inevitably inhibits us, but in doing so also opens up new capacities. By drawing on Deleuze's Nietzsche, I examine this ambiguity in relation to paranoia, and thus begin to approach an ethics that is capable of affirming this condition and productively utilizing it.

In Deleuze's view, *ressentiment* is one of Nietzsche's central concepts as it is at the heart of his conception of humanity. According to him, *ressentiment* is a condition in which one is unable to instinctively respond to an external stimulus, but consciously perceives it instead (1983, 111). Since *ressentiment* underlies our ability to feel, know and reflect on the world around us (and not just instinctively react to it), Nietzsche sees it as central to the development of human consciousness. '*Ressentiment* is not part of psychology,' Deleuze insists, 'but the whole of our psychology, without knowing it, is a part of *ressentiment*' (1983, 34). Deleuze further suggests that the men of *ressentiment* are *not* driven by an affirmative will to power, or affirmation, which seeks 'to affirm its difference' (1983, 78). Affirmation corresponds to an overflowing vital power that blindly strives for self-differentiation, and is, as such, akin to schizoid desiring-production. Instead, *ressentiment* is associated with the negative will to power. The latter wants 'to deny what differs' (Deleuze, ibid.), and is related to exhausted life, which seeks to oppose itself to self-differentiation of affirmative life and contain it, a tendency that brings it into line with repressive paranoia.

As in the case of paranoia, Deleuze insists that *ressentiment* is an illness, and not merely an emotional state. If paranoia arises when schizoid production invests the limits that interrupt it, *ressentiment* is the result of the malfunctioning force of forgetfulness, a force that is seen as beneficial by Nietzsche. This is so as this force refreshes the productive unconscious by freeing it from the investments made, and thus allows one to shake off the sense of obligation that arises from them. It is 'a plastic, regenerative and curative force' (Deleuze 1983, 113), which helps one to process the unconscious traces of past encounters and prevents their reaction to the new encounter from surfacing into consciousness. When this restorative force is impaired, the memories of past encounters are not processed by the unconscious, but instead rise into consciousness. As the memories of past encounters are seen as caused by the new encounter, one no longer responds to the latter, but gets caught up in conscious thought and memory. Instead of responding to the new encounter, one ends up reflecting on it.

Deleuze maintains that this structure, in which instinctive response is replaced by a conscious perception, is 'a formula which defines sickness in general' (1983, 114). He adds that 'Nietzsche is not simply saying that *ressentiment* is a sickness, but rather that sickness as such is a form of *ressentiment*' (ibid.). Every illness consists of us becoming conscious of the malfunctioning bodily processes that remain beneath our conscious perception when fully operative. Deleuze further maintains that *ressentiment* is characterized by the 'imputation of wrongs, the distribution of responsibilities, perpetual accusation' (1983, 118).[8] As it involves endless digestion of traces, which results in prolonged suffering, *ressentiment* manifests itself in a tendency to blame others for its suffering.[9] A man of *ressentiment*, suggests Deleuze, will 'feel the [affecting] object as a personal offence and affront because he makes the object responsible for his own powerlessness' to respond (1983, 118).

This repressive inclination directed toward the other, which, for Deleuze, paradigmatically manifests itself in the accusation 'It's your fault!', corresponds to the paranoiac tendency to police everyone who would disturb the boundaries that outline the invested order of things. The other repressive pole of paranoia, one directed toward one's own desiring-production, is framed by Nietzsche in terms of bad conscience, a condition that extends the operations of *ressentiment*. Like the latter, bad conscience is seen as an illness that fundamentally determines the character of humanity. According to Deleuze, bad conscience is constituted by 'turn[ing] back against itself' of the affirmative will to power, which is the same formulation used in *Anti-Oedipus* to characterize the self-regulation of paranoid desire. 'All the instincts that do not discharge themselves outwardly turn inward,' suggests Nietzsche, 'that is the origin of the "bad conscience"' (quoted in Deleuze 1983, 128). The genesis of bad conscience, which for Deleuze corresponds to the admission 'It's my fault!', further enhances human cognitive capacities. Nietzsche claims that it is due to the internalization of instincts that a human being acquires a rich and varied internal landscape (even if one haunted by guilt), and finally becomes 'an interesting animal' (2007, 16).

It is here that we can observe the ambiguity that so deeply characterizes Nietzsche's philosophy, and that can be observed also with his consideration of *ressentiment* and bad conscience. Nietzsche, who is frequently and intensely fascinated by a phenomenon a moment after he forcefully dismisses it, here stages the same turnaround. After declaring *ressentiment* and bad conscience to be devastating illnesses, he points to the advantageous effects of the latter. 'Illness,' Deleuze suggests

> separates me from what I can do . . . it narrows my possibilities and condemns me to a diminished milieu to which I can do no more than adapt myself. But, in another way, it reveals to me a new capacity, it endows me with a new will that I can make my own, going to the limit of a strange power (1983, 66).

According to Deleuze's account of Nietzsche, an illness, like a flu or a coronavirus, incapacitates us by inhibiting certain activities that we are no longer able to perform, but it also opens up strange vistas that were unavailable to us before. The paradigmatic examples of such ambivalent phenomena are *ressentiment* and bad conscience. The first illness inhibits the proto-human from being able to instinctively respond to stimuli (or even adequately – without being flooded by memories – engage with it at the level of consciousness), but at the same time develops capacities for conscious reflection. The evolution of the human mind, for Nietzsche, continues with bad conscience, through which 'basic ways of thinking have come into being, such as inferring, calculating, weighing and anticipating' (Ansell-Pearson 2007, xxii). As a result, he suggests that '[h]uman history would be altogether too stupid a thing without the spirit that the [sickly] have introduced into it' (Nietzsche 2007, 17).

Deleuze, consequently, suggests that diseases 'separate us from our power but at the same time they give us another power': they 'bring us new feelings and teach us new ways of being affected' (1983, 66). These new capacities to be affected reveal to us new, strange and even terrifying vistas. When reflecting on what meditation has taught him, Dominic Pettman suggests that 'one's deepest fears and anxieties live and breed in the invisible brine that exists in the fleeting, infinite space following the end of an exhalation, and before the next breath begins' (2020, 34). This disturbing feeling of being stuck between the inhale and the exhale is something that is very familiar to an asthmatic, who, during an asthma attack, has to put conscious effort into breathing. This experience, which, unless one practises meditation, remains utterly foreign to a healthy body, can be for Deleuze creatively exploited. He offers an analysis of such creative utilization in his *Essays Critical and Clinical* (1997), where he establishes a link between illness and literature. Deleuze's analysis focuses on how writers by means of literary activity bear witness to the extraordinary new vistas laid bare by their particular illnesses. In doing so, they not only diagnose their symptoms but are – by creatively engaging with them – even able to alleviate or transform them.

Ethics of paranoia

Similar to a disease, the COVID-19 restrictions (and the paranoid investments they induce) inhibit our powers, restrict our activity, and, as suggested by Deleuze above, narrow our possibilities by condemning us to a diminished milieu in which we can only adapt ourselves. To affirm this situation in which we find ourselves is to lean into the new possibilities afforded by it. Like in the case of *ressentiment* and asthma, where illness makes us aware of a certain malfunction, the formation of paranoiac investments, too, is accompanied by an expansion of consciousness. According to Deleuze and Guattari, 'there is no fixed subject unless there is repression' (1983, 26). In their view, a stable subjectivity is inevitably grounded in durable investments into a particular order of things, investments that are, thus, to a certain extent, paranoid.[10] For Deleuze (and Guattari), consciousness is not a site of genuine activity, and yet, since there is an affinity between paranoid investments and paranoid ways of thinking, we should acknowledge Sedgwick's recognition of the potential of the paranoid will to know. When she conceptualizes an alternative, *reparative* practice, she does not dismiss the paranoiac epistemology, but takes is as its starting point. In Sedgwick's view, 'the paranoid exigencies . . . are often necessary for nonparanoid knowing and utterance' (2003, 129). She adds that her activist friend's 'calm response . . . about the origins of HIV drew on a lot of research, her own and other people's, much of which required being paranoically structured' (ibid.).

Yet, in order to find a Deleuzian ethics that is able to cope with the COVID-19-induced paranoia, a different approach is needed. Deleuze, as noted above, maintains that every illness 'endows me with a new will that I can make my own, going to the limit of a strange power' (1983, 66). To expand on this new will which can be made my own, and consider it in relation to COVID-19, I engage with the ethical account that Deleuze presents in *The Logic of Sense*, a book published between *Nietzsche and Philosophy* and *Anti-Oedipus*. There he suggests that '[e]ither ethics has no sense at all, or this is what it means': 'to become worthy of what happens to us', or, as he restates it, 'to will the event' (1990, 169). To develop this ethical affirmation of the event, Deleuze draws inspiration from the French poet Joë Bousquet, who was severely wounded in the Second World War, and spent the rest of his life in constant pain, paralysed from his waist down, and confined to his bed. In spite of this dreadful accident, Bousquet was able to write: 'Become the man of your misfortunes; learn to embody their perfection and brilliance' (1990, 170). Through the literary activity provoked by his wound (which also features frequently in his poetic work) Bousquet was able to (re-)will the ill-fated event of his injury by giving it a new meaning and direction.

It is clear that Bousquet's outlook, which allowed him to become worthy of what happened to him, is completely incompatible with *ressentiment*. The emergence of the latter should indeed be seen as a failure to affirm the event. Deleuze makes this explicit when he suggests that to 'grasp whatever happens as unjust and unwarranted (it is always someone else's fault) is, on the contrary, what renders our sores repugnant – veritable *ressentiment*, the *ressentiment* of the event. There is no other ill will' (1990, 169). Harbouring resentfulness about one's illness, or a disastrous event such as the coronavirus outbreak, is for Deleuze a sign of ill will, one that is unable to will this event. A resentful attitude, which blames others for the catastrophic encounter, sees it as unjust, or seeks to reject the occurrence, points to an attachment to a particular order of things that was in place before the event took place. This attachment results in denying the change/difference brought about by this encounter, a trait that can be linked to both the negative will to power and paranoia.

It is important to note that for Deleuze resignation to, or even acceptance of, the event, should does not amount to affirmation. He elaborates on this fatalistic acceptance of what happens to us in *Nietzsche and Philosophy*, where he renders it as 'the yes of the ass' (1983, 182). The latter is related to an attitude that puts up with every assigned burden or responsibility and passively suffers through its misfortunes. Since it consists of a mere adaptation to the event, affirmation 'conceived of as acceptance, as affirmation of that which is', suggests Deleuze, 'is a false affirmation' (1990, 184). To fully affirm the event of the COVID-19 pandemic, and become worthy of it, would require a different orientation.

Substantiation of this orientation requires a clarification of Deleuze's notion of the event. Jon Roffe suggests that each event is linked to two ontologically distinct components, 'its ideality and its bodily actualization' (2020, 311). Strictly speaking, an event is a matter of ideality, which concerns the 'incorporeal' domain of meanings and ideas.[11] Yet, as such, it is inseparable from the domain of corporeality, which is one of material bodies and their causal encounters. Deleuze clarifies the relation between the two domains when he suggests that '[t]he event is not what occurs (an accident), it is inside what occurs, the purely expressed' (1990, 170). According to Deleuze, an event is expressed by, and thus associated with, the domain of encountering bodies, but cannot be reduced to this domain.

If I, for example, get hurt by a dear friend of mine, the way that this event is first expressed in me might be the feeling of hurt or anger toward them. Yet, after I, in a Spinozist manner, reflect on the circumstances that shaped this friend, and remind myself of the hardships that they endured, this event, i.e. its sense, could be construed differently, or, to put it Deleuze's terms, 'counter-actualized'. This counter-actualization could perhaps consist of my realization that their deed was not an intentional attempt to undermine me, but an inevitable outcome of their upbringing, which would allow me to face my friend in a more forgiving and constructive manner. Each bodily actualization, be it my response to my friend's hurtful deed, or the bullet passing through Bousquet's spine, is thus always open to being counter-actualized in a new and different way.

To will an event, therefore, as Roffe aptly sums up, amounts to 'an act of the will that affirms the event in its excess over any given actualization' (2020, 307). This ethical orientation, which consists of modifying our relationship to what happens, is precisely what is at stake in the above-mentioned example of illness. Willing an illness cannot take place if one merely accepts the suffering it gives rise to, but has to include finding ways to productively mobilize the changes it brings about. To give a more trivial example, to will a hangover is to go beyond feeling sorry for oneself or having a bad conscience for having drunk that much, but to affirmatively engage, perhaps, in an exploration of certain kinds of music, the ones that our bodies are more receptible to while slowed down and inhibited in this way. Finally, the same kind of ethical reorientation can be adopted for an event of the magnitude of the coronavirus pandemic. The latter has disrupted our lives in countless ways. Yet, to be able to will this terrible disruption, we need to find to a new, more empowering relation to these changes, thus giving it a new meaning. This is achieved by being able to counter-actualize not only lockdowns, curfews, social distancing measures and other prescribed limitations that we came to paranoidly invest, but also potential COVID-19 infections, thus exploiting what they make possible for us.

Once more citing Bousquet, Deleuze beautifully glosses the power of this ethical approach when he suggests that it ultimately allows us to 'assign to plagues, tyrannies, and the most frightful wars the comic possibility of having reigned for nothing' (1990, 151). Plagues, tyrannies and wars are happenings of the gravest kind, events that are difficult to see as anything other than disastrous. Yet, if one is able to grasp these events in a different way and move beyond the terror that they inspire in us, all their unbearable heaviness becomes comically ineffective. The point that Deleuze is making is that not even the most tyrannical despot, with all his power and might, is prevented from appearing as eternally glorious in the eyes of history. 'There's nothing that anyone can ever do to reduce the meaning of a word, an act, or a life, to just one thing,' suggests Roffe, 'despite their seriousness, tyrants have only ever been clowns' (2020, 311). It is up to us, then, to push beyond our *ressentiment*, acquiescence and all the '*if only*'s that this pandemic has inspired, and invent ways of living that will allow us to face its consequences with lightness or even laughter. This is obviously easier said than done. In fact, achieving this seems to border on impossible, but, as Spinoza rightly reminds us, all 'things excellent are as difficult as they are rare' (2002, 382).

Notes

1 The translated collection of Agamben's interventions can be found at https://aphelis.net/agamben-coronavirus-pandemic-interventions (accessed: 21 August 2021).

2 It has to be noted that schizoprenia as a productive process should not be confused with schizophrenia as illness. Deleuze and Guattari repeatedly stress that schizophrenic illness arises only when schizophrenia as a process is forcefully stalled or prolonged. Such interruption of the desiring-production is also conductive of other linesses, such as neurosis, perversion and, ultimately, paranoia.

3 Deleuze and Guattari suggest that capitalism is initiated by a conjunction of two *decoded* (i.e. unregulated) flows, namely, 'the flow of free capital (i.e., money not bound by State regulation) and the flow of so-called free or "naked" labour (i.e, labour power not owed in advance to the State through either slavery or serfdom)' (Roffe 2000, 107). Roffe claims that this first conjunction should be understood as 'the general matrix for the situation of capitalism' as it sets off the dramatic unravelling of fixed belief systems enforced by the despotic state, a process that is central to the functioning of capitalism (ibid.).

4 Read adds that axioms 'relate to no other scene or sphere, such as religion, politics or law, which would provide their ground or justification' (2008, 145).

5 According to Canetti, the despot and the paranoiac are 'one and the same' (1981, 447).

6 Deleuze and Guattari insist that 'it is not machines that have created capitalism, but capitalism that creates machines' (1983, 233). In their view, it is the realization of profit that drives technological innovation, which disrupts the established ways of acting and thinking.

7 Bette Midler's tweet stating that 'it started out as a virus and mutated into an IQ test' might be paradigmatic of such attitudes (available at: https://twitter.com/BetteMidler/status/1425250648283566080 (accessed 26 August 2021).

8 This once again aligns *ressentiment* with paranoia, as the latter exhibits 'mania for finding causal relations' (Canetti 1981, 452).

9 Deleuze proposes that the 'man of *ressentiment* in himself is a being full of pain: the sclerosis or hardening of his consciousness, the rapidity with which every excitation sets and freezes within him, the weight of the traces that invade him are so many cruel sufferings' (1983, 116.).

10 In the absence of paranoid investments, our psychic life is subject to an ongoing revolution, where no impression or belief is permanent, but, to put it in Nietzsche's terms, is immediately subject to erasure by the forces of forgetfulness.

11 For events as incorporeal see Deleuze 1990, 4–5.

References

Agamben, G. (2020), 'The Invention of an Epidemic', *European Journal of Psychoanalysis*. Available online: http://www.journal-psychoanalysis.eu/coronavirus-and-philosophers (accessed 26 August 2021).

Ansell-Pearson, K. (2007), 'Introduction: on Nietzsche's critique of morality', in Nietzsche, F. *On the Genealogy of Morality*, ed. Keith Ansell-Pearson, trans. Carol Diethe, Cambridge: Cambridge University Press.

Bauer, M. and Tomažin, A. (2017), 'The Only Thing I Would Impose is Fragmentation: An Interview with Nick Land', *Synthetic Zero*. Available online: https://syntheticzero.net/2017/06/19/the-only-thing-i-would-impose-is-fragmentation-an-interview-with-nick-land/ (accessed 26 August 2021).

Bratton, B. (2021), *The Revenge of the Real: Politics for a Post-pandemic World*, London: Verso, ebook.

Canetti, E. (1981), *Crowds and Power*, trans. Carol Stewart, New York: Continuum.

Deleuze, D (1971), 'Codes, Capitalism, Flows, Decoding Flows, Capitalism and Schizophrenia, Psychoanalysis', *The Deleuze Seminars*. Available online: https://deleuze.cla.purdue.edu/seminars/anti-oedipus-i/lecture-01 (accessed 10 August 2021).

Deleuze, G. (1983), *Nietzsche and Philosophy*, trans. Hugh Tomlinson, New York: Columbia University Press.

Deleuze, G. (1990), *The Logic of Sense*, ed. Constantin V. Boundas, trans. Mark Lester and Charles Stivale, New York: Columbia University Press.

Deleuze, G. (1997), *Essays Critical and Clinical*, trans. Daniel W. Smith and Michael A. Greco, Minneapolis: University of Minnesota Press, pp. 138–151.

Deleuze, G. and Guattari, F. (1983), *Anti-Oedipus: Capitalism and Schizophrenia*, trans. Robert Hurley, Mark Seem, and Helen R. Lane, Minneapolis: University of Minnesota Press.

Houellebecq, M. (2000), *Atomised*, trans. Frank Wynne, London: Vintage.

Houellebecq, M. (2005), *The Possibility of an Island*, trans. Gavin Bowd, London: Weidenfeld & Nicholson.

Houellebecq, M. (2011), *The Map and the Territory*, trans. Gavin Bowd, London: Heinemann.

Jameson, F. (1988), 'Cognitive Mapping', in Nelson, C. and Grossberg, L. (eds.) *Marxism and the Interpretation of Culture*, London: Macmillan, pp. 347–360.

Kosofsky Sedgwick, E. (2003), 'Paranoid Reading and Reparative Reading, or, You're So Paranoid, You Probably Think This Essay Is About You', in *Touching Feeling: Affect, Pedagogy, Performativity*, Durham: Duke University Press, pp. 123–151.

Marx K. and Engels, F. (1848), 'Manifesto of the Communist Party', *Marxists Internet Archive*. Available online: http://www.marxists.org/archive/marx/works/1848/communist-manifesto/ch01.htm (accessed 26 August 2021).

Nietzsche, F. (2007), *On the Genealogy of Morality*, ed. Keith Ansell-Pearson, trans. Carol Diethe, Cambridge: Cambridge University Press.
Pettman, D. (2020), *The Humid Condition*, Santa Barbara: Punctum Books.
Read, J. (2008), 'The Age of Cynicism: Deleuze and Guattari on Production of Subjectivity in Capitalism', in Buchanan, I. (ed.) *Deleuze and Politics*, Edinburgh: Edinburgh University Press, pp. 139–159.
Roffe, J. (2000), *Abstract Market Theory*, London: Palgrave Macmillan.
Roffe, J. (2020), *The Works of Gilles Deleuze I: 1953–1969*, Melbourne: re-press.
Sarasin, P. (2020), 'Understanding the Coronavirus with Foucault?', *Genealogy+Critique*. Available online: https://blog.genealogy-critique.net/essays/254/understanding-corona-with-foucault (accessed 10 August 2021).
Spinoza, B. (2002), *Ethics*, in Morgan, M. L. (ed), *Spinoza: Complete Works*, trans. Samuel Shirley, Indianapolis: Hackett, pp. 213–382.
WHO. (2020), 'Managing the COVID-19 Infodemic: Promoting Healthy Behaviours and Mitigating the Harm from Misinformation and Disinformation', *World Health Organization*. Available online: https://www.who.int/news/item/23-09-2020-managing-the-covid-19-infodemic-promoting-healthy-behaviours-and-mitigating-the-harm-from-misinformation-and-disinformation (accessed 22 August 2021).

12

Thinking the COVID-19 as an Event: A Physical and Spiritual Illness in the Post-Truth Era

Francisco J. Alcalá[1]

Gilles Deleuze and Félix Guattari posed the need for a milieu of immanence as a material condition for the emergence and survival of philosophy, which in the origins of the discipline corresponded to the society of 'free and equal friends/rivals' that was the Greek polis, and nowadays to the equivalence in the commodity-form imposed by global capitalism (1994, 97–98). Therefore, the epistemological and political task of philosophical thought consists – now as then – in introducing a new order or a strictly immanent selection into that milieu, banishing the threats of both transcendence and relativism (Deleuze 1998, 136–137).

These issues are gaining renewed relevance in the context of the COVID-19 global pandemic that we have been experiencing since the beginning of 2020. Although far from enabling philosophical thought to survive, the rise of contagion as a new milieu of immanence seems to certify its decline: public interventions on the subject made by some philosophers have been harshly criticized, mainly for giving free rein to their own obsessions and frivolously subsuming the new problems brought about by the pandemic into those previously posed by their respective 'trademark' philosophies. This is so in the case of Giorgio Agamben (2020), whose approach has confused the essential healthcare work of states in the face of a health emergency with the threat of a new state of emergency, leading Slavoj Žižek (2020) to ironically title one of the chapters in his book on the pandemic 'Monitor and Punish, Yes Please!' As an author, Žižek, who has also been criticized for envisioning in the pandemic the advent of communism, has performed a remarkable exercise of theoretical boldness – and probably also of editorial opportunism – that seems to replace the old-fashioned owl of Minerva by the charter flight, more in keeping with the times.

In this chapter, I aim to demonstrate that, in this context of the discrediting of philosophy (Diéguez 2020), Deleuze and Guattari's thought can help us to undertake the task of philosophically addressing the pandemic in its event dimension, which involves both physical and spiritual 'symptoms' that demand to be counter-effectuated in an ethical and political response.

Prelude: what is an event?

When we try to form a more or less spontaneous idea of an event, we usually find its everyday meaning, which is no less profound for that. Thus, for any of us, an event is always 'something' that takes place without our being able to foresee or explain it: a special kind of 'happening' that interrupts the 'natural' – i.e. expected – course of occurrences. Therefore, there is a quotidian sense of the event, according to which it is always that paradoxical logic that governs the unprecedented or the untimely in the real; that which should not take place and yet it has.

Deleuze's philosophy gives a remarkable consistency to the concept of event, considered by the author as the core notion of his thought (1995, 141, 143). The key to understanding the event lies in the implicit definition of the concept contained in *Difference and Repetition*, which is a book focused on a different problem: that of the foundation of thought. Deleuze considers that thought must renounce the foundation when it is transcendent; that is to say, external to the founded reality. This is why he proposes that the foundation of individuals must be interior or immanent to them (1994, 246, 249–250). Thus, the 'atoms' whose changing distributions generate individuals are the new 'ground' of reality, and Deleuze calls them 'pre-individual singularities' or 'individuating differences'. Consequently, individuals are nothing more than a simulation or a by-product of those distributions of singularities that constitute the ontology proper (Zourabichvili 2012, 117).

But what is the place of the event in this approach? Deleuze distinguishes three temporalities or syntheses of time that constitute the three forms of repetition (1994, 94): a physical repetition in habit (living present), a metaphysical repetition in Memory (pure past) and an ontological repetition in the eternal return (future). The first synthesis constitutes a 'pretension' of every individual – persisting, the second one deepens this pretension towards a virtual object that acts as its foundation, the third one undoes every individual and every foundation to restart the process again on new foundations. And the event finds the temporality that is proper to it in the third synthesis (89; Lapoujade 2014, 79). It follows that the third synthesis produces a new distribution of pre-individual reality (the ontological-transcendental or 'virtual'), which entails the reconfiguration of the individuated reality that we are and with which we relate (the empirical or 'actual'). And if the eternal return concerns pure events, it is because the event is precisely that redistribution of the pre-individual singularities that makes up the ontological-transcendental (Deleuze 1994, 246; 1990, 51–52; Lapoujade 2014, 64) – not for nothing, the third synthesis is 'dialectical', and dialectics is the science of problems or pure events (Deleuze 1990, 8; 1994, 188).

Deleuze, therefore, suggests that the event is a redistribution that forces us to ask ourselves: 'What has happened?' (1990, series 22). This is the question about the event that – silent and inexorable – has taken place behind our backs, redistributing the powers that constitute us or displacing one problem for the benefit of another so that everything will have changed once again.

Hence, in *Difference and Repetition*, the event refers to the logical principle of the redistribution of pre-individual singularities at the virtual level, which transforms the actual or individuated reality and gives rise to the new. Thus, it mediates our relation with reality as a transcendental field and establishes a new way of thinking about the individuals, which relates each individual reality rather with a constituent other than with the pure identity of a fixed essence. Therefore, the vicissitudes of Deleuze's technical concept do not overlook the quotidian – but profound – sense of the event to which I referred above.

The COVID-19 as an event: what has happened?

If, as we have just seen, an event is a redistribution of the constitutive powers of reality at the transcendental level that leads to a more or less drastic change in the empirical reality where our individual existence unfolds, we cannot but recognize that the COVID-19 pandemic constitutes a particularly exceptional event in our times.

The pandemic outbreak has been a paradoxical situation in itself, insofar as it has combined the unpredictable with the expected, as warned for decades by the scientific community – and even by a science fiction film by Steven Soderbergh: *Contagion*. In this sense, the possibility of a new pandemic of global impact that was announced in the epidemics finally contained – bird flu (2009), Ebola (2014–2016), Zika virus (2015–present) – as well as in the swine flu or H1N1 pandemic (2009–2010), and of course in the AIDS pandemic (1981–present), ended up being realized in a new coronavirus spread from animals to humans, or rather, from other animals to human animals. And if it is true that there are 'critical points of the event' analogous to the boiling or melting points of matter, which determine whether or not a given event takes place (Deleuze 1990, 80), this time these have been determined by the virulence of the physical spread of the disease and the increased mortality that it has shown.

After the crisis and in the face of the spread of the disease, states were forced to activate a biopolitical machinery that we thought was a thing of the past, whose screeching was hurting the ears of citizens accustomed to the fluid freedom that in today's control societies is synchronized with the rhythm of consumption. We then experience the 'spiritual' effects that the pandemic has brought to no lesser extent, mainly associated with another type of infection: that of opinion in times of post-truth.

Following the above, it is worth asking what the COVID-19 event has been about, i.e. how everyday reality has been redistributed as a result of its unpredictable – but expected – shake-up?

Explicitly or implicitly, most authors who have dealt with the pandemic philosophically have echoed its character as an event. Among these approaches, it is worth highlighting the latest lucid text by anthropologist David Graeber, entitled 'After the Pandemic, We Can't Go Back to Sleep' (2020), which approaches the COVID-19 pandemic as if it were the awakening from a dream that has changed our awareness of everyday reality – a dream to which we cannot return once the threat of the disease has dissipated. Also noteworthy is Bruno Latour's approach in his latest book, *Où suis-je? Leçons du confinement à l'usage des terrestres* [Where Am I? Lessons from Confinement for Terrestrial Inhabitants] (2021), which takes as a model the experience of the protagonist of Kafka's *Metamorphosis* – who also wakes up from a dream, but transformed into a cockroach – to address the experience of the pandemic.

And the truth is that this awakening from a dream in which everything is upside down is a good metaphor for what has happened in this pandemic. Each one of us can make the mental experiment of remembering the first weeks after the declaration of the pandemic by the WHO on 11 March 2020 and the implementation of the restrictions by the public authorities through biopolitical machinery without precedent in this century. We woke up starring in a strange science fiction film – or even a fantastic film – in which everyday reality had become enigmatic and dangerous: we knew little about the disease caused by the new coronavirus, about the terrible consequences that could result from contracting it, or about the mechanisms through which the contagion – that was proving to be very high given the data – was produced. Everyday gestures that form the backbone of interpersonal relationships, such as hugging or shaking hands, and even seeing each other's faces, now hidden under the obligatory mask, had become reckless and even obscene. Daily activities essential for subsistence such as shopping or going to work in the case of 'essential activities' had become an extreme sport that exposed us to contagion and from which we returned uneasy, striving to ward off the spectre of disease through compulsive disinfection. Nothing was as we knew it overnight.

Therefore, it is possible to accept the thesis that I stated at the beginning about the emergence of contagion, on the occasion of the pandemic event, as a new milieu of immanence that 'equalizes' us all, in the same way as does the commodity-form of globalized capitalism or the society of free and equal friends of Greek democracy – and the truth is that, far from being opposed to the former, the new milieu of immanence is sustained on them. Virtually all of us are COVID-19 patients or carriers, and there we are hence on the same plane of immanence, which must serve as a principle for thinking about the phenomenon. We must start from there, from the universalization of contagion, to establish the new distinctions, practices and concepts that will make this desert habitable again – a desert that we can't renounce, since, as Deleuze's thought teaches, it is the desert of Being or the real. So let us start from this equalization in contagion in our approach to the pandemic, a new transcendental field of thought in this event in which we find ourselves caught up. What does this terrible possibility of falling ill and dying, elevated to the most immediate universality, teach us?

Readers of Deleuze know that, in his philosophy, contagion presents a strictly immanent or 'horizontal' logic that is linked to the earth, which is the logic of the rhizome from *A Thousand Plateaus* and, ultimately, that of the disjunctive synthesis of *Difference and Repetition* (Deleuze and Guattari 2004, 6; Deleuze 1994, 41–42; 1990, 179–180). Being is a desert that supports different distributions without reducing itself to any of them; that is to say, opposing an 'inertial' resistance to any attempt to establish a definitive distribution (Deleuze 1995, 146). In other words, the rhizome or disjunctive synthesis is the immanent logic that flattens, redistributes and mixes everything at the level of Being that is by nature univocal or non-compartmentalized. To this extent, it opposes the compartmentalization of Being or its definitive distribution, which always takes place at the expense of the pure immanence of Being, by asserting an external – 'transcendent' – criterion. This compartmentalization, operated by the judgement of attribution, responds to a transcendent or 'vertical' logic that makes the virtual pass into actual existence on the condition that its reality is denaturalized, imposing artificial and therefore always provisional distributions on it.

But let us return to contagion: our societies are built on all kinds of artificial distributions or hierarchies, whose arbitrariness perpetuates inequalities, injustices and grievances that afflict human animals, non-human animals, and even the planet Earth. So while we will not go so far as to speak of an 'apology for contagion' (Alba Rico 2020), we will affirm that valuable lessons can be drawn from it to continue with life and thought on the face of earth once the rigours of the globalized disease allow us to do so. Contagion disproves the given reality once and for all and encourages us to rethink and transform it, i.e. it encourages us to distribute the given reality differently. Contagion also leads to a rethinking of individual identity in an era of closing borders and exclusionary nationalism, relating it to the vicinity of a constituent other rather than to an identity established beforehand through an external instance such as essence (national, ethnic, political, gender, etc.).

In this sense, Jean-Luc Nancy identified contagion with com-passion, defining it as: 'The contact of being with one another in this turmoil. Compassion is not altruism, nor is it identification; it is the disturbance of violent relatedness' (1995, XIII). The first experience that follows from contagion is thus that of being-with or contiguity and, ultimately, the experience of interdependence. We necessarily exist in common with other human beings, non-human animals, and the planet Earth. Therefore, our existence depends on the existence of other humans and, to no lesser extent, on that of the rest of the earth's inhabitants and the very survival of the planet in conditions conducive to the development of life.

In his last book published during his lifetime, *Un trop humain virus* (An All Too Human Virus) (2020), Nancy himself made a fundamental distinction concerning the disease that is shaking the world: while in the past most diseases were exogenous or independent of human action, recent epidemics and pandemics are endogenous or the direct consequence of human action. This seems to be the case for SARS-CoV-2 and, in general, for the other coronaviruses that affect our species (HCoV) and cause infection also in animals. It is, therefore, a 'zoonotic' disease, i.e. it is a disease that can be transmitted from animals to humans and is probably of animal origin. Not for nothing did the first report of COVID-19 come from health authorities in the Chinese city of Wuhan, who linked twenty-seven cases of pneumonia of unknown aetiology to common exposure to a wholesale market of seafood, fish and other live animals in the city (Spanish Ministry of Health 2021). The way we humans treat the animals we consume, their ecosystems and the planet in general undoubtedly has an impact on the life of this *homo sapiens* who believe they are dissociated from the environment that surrounds them and reduces the other things that exist to *Bestand* (stock).

Recognizing this does not imply that we should accept the invariably stupid discourse that the pandemic is an act of revenge taken by Nature – with a capital letter – against the excesses of human beings, their *hybris*, appealing to a theological-moral narrative to explain an infinitely more complex phenomenon and bordering on justifying the humanitarian tragedy of the disease through supposed collective guilt. Nor does it imply accepting the 'whitewashing' of what has happened with symmetrically inverse stupidity, which leads to disregarding the warnings of specialists and precedents to exempt human beings from all responsibility, shielding their current way of life and once again entrusting the way out of the crisis solely to technology ('Once the dog has been vaccinated – from the borders inwards, watch out – rabies is over' . . . for the moment).[2]

At this point, we should not disregard Badiou's idea (2020), according to which the emergence of the COVID-19 pandemic follows from two intersections: an intersection of nature with human society (we know that bats carry a wide variety of coronaviruses and the genetic origin of SARS-CoV-2 leads to these animals, and we also have information about the poor sanitary conditions of the Wuhan animal market: Spanish Ministry of Health 2021), and an intersection of the current globalization, which has enabled the rapid global spread of the virus, with the archaic hygiene measures that characterize this type of animal market.

Anyway, it follows that there is a 'contagion' that is constitutive of the human species – the most collaborative of all primates (Diéguez 2020) – and arguably of life on earth itself, at the basis of the terrible contagion that worries us today. The event of the pandemic that causes the second one makes us aware of the first one. And we also become aware that there is probably no better way to ward off future manifestations of this pathological contagion than to take care of our constitutive contagion, i.e. our contiguity and interdependence with other human beings, non-human animals, and the planet Earth. If the experience of pathological contagion awakens the immunitary individual from their dream of immunity, the experience of contiguity or constitutive 'contagion' awakens the individual from their immunitary dream. The pandemic event thus brings us back to the ecological experience of the planetary community, which is not exclusively human. Humans cannot survive alone, but neither can we survive with our backs turned to non-human animals and the planet Earth.

Therefore, the individual does not emerge unscathed from the pandemic event. The COVID-19 actualizes the milieu of immanence of global capitalism in the universal possibility of contagion, revealing in addition both the interdependence and the vulnerability of human lives (Badiou 2020) – in relation both to the lives of other human beings and to the ecological niche that hosts them. And this rediscovered vulnerability also has socio-political and economic consequences. It makes us aware – again: awakens us – of the nonsense in which economic and social relations are embedded, which until now seemed so reasonable to us. This sudden realization is certainly consistent with Deleuze's assertion that there is a subjective mutation correlated with the event that leads to perceiving as intolerable what was hitherto quotidian (2007, 234). Graeber puts it brilliantly:

> In reality, the crisis we just experienced was waking from a dream, a confrontation with the actual reality of human life, which is that we are a collection of fragile beings taking care of one another, and that those who do the lion's share of this care work that keeps us alive are overtaxed, underpaid, and daily humiliated, and that a very large proportion of the population don't do anything at all but spin fantasies, extract rents, and generally get in the way of those who are making, fixing, moving, and transporting things, or tending to the needs of other living beings. It is imperative that we not slip back into a reality where all this makes some sort of inexplicable sense, the way senseless things so often do in dreams (Graeber 2020).

Therefore, the COVID-19 pandemic makes us experience the nonsense of a large part of the hierarchies on which our routines, movements, relationships, expectations and, in the end, our lives are based. Isolated from the inertia that underpins their daily lives, confined individuals realize the senselessness of spending so much time away from home working while paying someone else to look after their children or investing more time in building one's CV than one's biography. They also realize the value of care work – at home, in hospitals, schools, nursing homes, etc. – and the importance of public services such as health and education, which so many voices used to denigrate in the name of the neoliberal dogma of private management and tax cuts . . . We realize that even to the point of valuing the service to the general interest provided by the postman, the haulier or the shop assistant. We end up thus, as happened in Spain, going out onto the balcony every evening to applaud the health workers who care for the sick at the risk of their lives while the rest of us are confined – at least, those of us who can. And we realize, in the end, that perhaps the disposition of reality and, among it, that of the life projects and expectations that we have – assembled around the 'promises' of an economy that is ultimately indifferent to our well-being – do not make as much sense as we had imagined, captivated by the dream from which we have just awakened and into which we will probably fall again when the situation has normalized. It is certainly not a good sign that the noise of petty political debate, if not outright hate speech, has replaced that of applause.

Finally, I will consider the 'spiritual' symptoms of the global phenomenon that COVID-19 is, from the point of view of its origin in the aporias that the 'return' of biopolitics – confinements, curfews . . . – entails as an unexpected brake on the fluidity of control societies (Deleuze 1995, 177–182), as well as from the point of view of current post-truth dynamics.

Foucault placed disciplinary societies between the eighteenth century and the beginning of the twentieth century, when they would have reached their splendour and then ceded their hegemony to control societies. In both cases, it is a model of social domination, albeit built on different social and technological foundations. Disciplinary societies are characterized by confinement, which makes the individual pass throughout their life through different institutions that exercise a form of sovereignty over them: they thus exercise their power over life through confinement in the hospital, school, barracks, prison, etc. However, with the deepening of democracy, the increasing consolidation of individual freedom and the development of digital technologies, these disciplinary societies that 'moulded' individuals by confining them to institutions are giving way to control societies, which exercise their dominion over individuals through more sophisticated techniques that make it possible to manage life in an open space. As Deleuze eloquently explains, there is a shift from an economic model based on moulded currency and factory labour to one based on fluctuating exchanges and office work, which 'modulates' individuals – that is, continuously moulds them in space and time – with devices such as merit-based wages, teleworking and continuous learning (178, 180).

It follows from this brief description that many of the 'spiritual' symptoms brought about by the pandemic are due to an unexpected return of some of the biopolitical methods that characterized disciplinary societies within today's control societies:

confinement, curfews, mobility restrictions, etc. These are mechanisms based on confinement to whose limitations the contemporary individual is not accustomed. Not for nothing did Deleuze note that the two societies had two very different juridical ways of life and that the recent transition from one to the other was already a source of hesitation in the law of the time (179). Anyway, we can at best speak of a return of some of the characteristic elements of disciplinary societies in today's control societies, but we can by no means speak of a regression towards the former. On the contrary, state management of the pandemic confirms Deleuze's description of control societies on a global level at every point: the empire of digital numbers (*chiffre*) that determine access to information (180), the control mechanisms that determine at every moment the position of an individual in an open environment (181), or Félix Guattari's fantasy of an electronic card that would allow us to move freely by opening a series of barriers . . . until it was subject to temporary or permanent restrictions, carried out in the so-called 'COVID passport' (181–182). It also confirms his intuition about a new medicine 'without doctors and patients', but with carriers ('potential patients' and transmitters) and 'risk subjects' to be controlled (182).

In this situation, there is in our societies a diversity of reactive responses to health measures taken by governments, marked by two dominant tendencies that are at home under cover of post-truth. On the one hand, there is a proliferation of those who are unjustifiably sceptical and rebellious against the advances in knowledge of COVID-19 and the health measures adopted by governments, just because they suppose that – in case they are mistaken and get sick – they will not get the worst of it thanks to their socio-economic status, relative youth or good general health. On the other hand, there is also a certain 'fear of freedom' in some sectors, mostly progressives, which welcome almost any new restriction adopted by governments – when they do not openly demand it. They perhaps have in common the misunderstanding of the meaning of legitimate freedom; the former confuse it with a childish form of agency, the latter with an immunitary withdrawal into individual security and convictions under the pretext of the common good.

Thus, it must be acknowledged that – as Adorno warned – opinion can also be infected, and its speed of expansion or contagion in this crisis does not lag behind that of the virus: we, therefore, speak of an 'infodemic' that runs parallel to the pandemic. Consequently, it is possible to affirm, with Taylor Shelton (2020), that we are facing the first post-truth pandemic in history.

While post-truth theorists often appeal to 'objective facts' to combat it (McIntyre 2018), both the negationism of COVID-19 and the desire for authoritarianism seem to prove Bruno Latour was right when he stated in a recent interview that a fact without cultural background is a lamb among wolves (Latour 2020). It is useless to wield scientific facts in a cultural context whose ideological and/or emotional obfuscation offers them no support and flatly refuses to accept them. Furthermore, theorists such as Lee McIntyre, when he states that 'these critics were missing the point of what science was really about: engaging facts rather than values' referring to the post-structuralists (2018, 130), overlook at least two important issues.

The first issue was already pointed out by Descartes when he indicated that it is typical of *esprits malsains* (sick minds) to intend to conduct themselves in the world of life with a certainty similar to that provided by science (1999, 359). Translated into this context, we could put it this way: scientific facts do not offer unambiguous guidelines for articulating a life project following them so that when we are involved in the world of life and are people as well as scientists, it is inevitable that we also commit ourselves to values. This, I repeat, makes us people, not outmoded metaphysicians or relativists conjured against truth. Nietzsche becomes more topical in this respect, and with him Deleuze once again, because affirmative values, devoid of resentment and oriented towards the common good – which we could qualify in political terms as 'republican', following Pérez Tapias (2020) – are those that will make it possible to elaborate a consistent narrative that does not succumb to the narcissistic and self-serving temptation of post-truth that delegitimizes the available scientific evidence on COVID-19, envisages implausible international conspiracies or identifies the health measures adopted by governments with a re-edition of the totalitarian state. Therefore, we need to build a narrative or a cultural background for scientific facts so that they can be taken into account in the formation of public opinion and democratic decision-making without succumbing to scientism dogmatism or, of course, to the damaging relativistic influence of post-truth.

The second issue that McIntyre's approach neglects is that, rather than with scientific facts, ordinary citizens relate to data that are presented to them as having this epistemological status. In other words, we generally do not have direct access to scientific facts, but rather to their representation in the form of the data offered to us by science, science communicators and an endless number of falsifiers who want to pass off their information as scientific, using social networks, the web or the media to circulate it at a global level. This distinction makes it possible to understand that post-truth cannot be fought against by wielding only scientific facts independently of the cultural background that allows people to decide between data claiming such a status. In an interesting and well-documented article, Shelton shows how data alone is not only no antidote to post-truth, but that post-truth itself is based on data-centred societies:

> It's evident that coronavirus has revealed not only the general inadequacy of our data infrastructures and assemblages, but also the more general shift towards a 'post-truth' disposition in contemporary social life, wherein 'objective facts are less influential in shaping public opinion than appeals to emotion and personal belief' (Oxford Dictionaries, 2016) ... But ... It would be a mistake to see the centrality of data as being somehow the opposite from the larger post-truth apparatus that leads data and facts to exist on unstable ground. Instead, these two ostensibly opposed dynamics are fundamentally intertwined and co-produced (Shelton 2020, 2).

It is thus paradoxical that the production, analysis and consumption of data on COVID-19 during the pandemic have not improved the objective knowledge of the virus and the disease it causes in the wider society. In this respect, the founder of the COVID Tracking Project said: 'The point is that every country's numbers are the result of a specific set of testing and accounting regimes. Everyone is cooking the data, one way or another. And yet . . . people continue to rely on charts showing different numbers' (Madrigal 2020). Thus, we can conclude that it is partly this hegemony of data, the representation of the desired 'naked' fact, which gives free rein to its distortion to favour the circulation of post-truth. Much is said about the manipulation by governments and private institutions to serve their interests, but 'the less commented upon dynamic is how these actions remain cloaked in the veneer of being data-driven and scientifically grounded even as the actions and ends to which they are put are anything but' (Shelton 2020, 2).

Conclusion: politics of the event or how to be at the height of what happens to us?

In Deleuze and Guattari's philosophy, the logical sequence of socio-political change sets out the political challenge that the event proposes to us. First, there is an event as an act or an incorporeal transformation that goes unnoticed and extracts an assemblage of enunciation that realizes it – 'workers of the world, unite!' (Deleuze and Guattari 2004, 83). Second, this event-assemblage gives rise to a new subjectivity that establishes equally new relations with all spheres of life, removing itself from the power relations and forms of knowledge of the present assemblage, so that what used to be quotidian becomes intolerable (Deleuze 2007, 234). Finally, there is the need to 'counter-effectuate' the event; that is, to create new assemblages or lifestyles that respond to the new subjectivity, placing individuals and societies at the height of what is happening to them. It is in these unprecedented assemblages where the subjectivity that inspired them by anticipating their forms will be reinserted.

Therefore, it is also necessary to be at the height of the event that this illness is – to counter-effectuate it – by responding to its physical and 'spiritual' effects through the constitution of new assemblages. I conclude this chapter by offering some thoughts on the subject.

First, I should point out the need to address our constitutive interdependence at the social, political and ecological levels by establishing international solidarity agreements, effective public policies and interpersonal care networks. Trying to reverse such a global and interpersonal situation like this pandemic on an exclusively local and institutional level would be useless, as well as unsupportive. We must also resist the hate speeches that attribute a nationality to the virus and its variants to pose the problem in terms of a war of nations, and understand that immanence in contagion makes us today more than ever citizens of the world; that is, citizens of the planet Earth and fellow travellers of the other beings that inhabit it and of the planet itself. Only in this way will we be prepared to overcome the ecological crisis that is looming, of which the COVID-19 crisis is probably only a prelude.

Second, it is necessary to realize the political upheaval that the event entails and understand the affirmative role of the health measures adopted in this crisis context. In trying to be critical of state powers and the use of biopolitics, we should not end up supporting a genocidal 'thanatopolitics' also exercised by states in the name of safeguarding the economy and assuming an unbearable human cost (Pérez Tapias

2020). We must understand, in short, that after the upheaval brought about by such an event, biopolitics may well take on an affirmative role, just as Žižek intelligently notes that 'not to shake hands and isolate when needed is today's form of solidarity' (2020, 77).

Third, and finally, faced with the double danger of post-truth and of its critics using it as a Trojan horse to reintroduce the most superficial neo-positivism into contemporary thought, it is necessary to realize the importance of posing problems, of establishing a solvent narrative that cannot be neutral as a dike to contain infodemics and its undesirable socio-political consequences. Without a cultural background of widespread trust in science that recognizes the provisionality of the explanations ('truths') it offers us, as do virtually all those who have taken an interest in the way scientific disciplines evolve, any hesitation on the part of scientists in their theories and predictions will be perceived as a sign of relativism that will arouse the distrust of the scientific enterprise and lead to the nefarious pursuit of conspiracy theories and 'alternative facts' – and in this pandemic, there have been many such hesitations due to the logical lack of knowledge about the disease and the hasty publication of preprints that had not yet passed peer review. In short, dogmatism is undesirable even when it supports a correct cause, such as science. That is why I argue that it is necessary here to redirect the counter-effectuation in the assemblage towards a promotion of scientific and humanistic culture focused on the formulation of problems, which does not fall into any 'dogmatic image of thought' – be it anti-scientific or technocratic.

Note

1 Francisco J. Alcalá is a postdoctoral researcher at the University of Granada, currently on a two-year postdoctoral fellowship at the University of Barcelona (Margarita Salas programme). He carries out his research in the Aporía Group of the University of Barcelona and the Project of the Spanish Ministry of Science, Innovation and Universities 'La mirada filosófica como mirada médica' (The Philosophical Gaze as a Medical Gaze) —PGC2018-094253-B-I00—. Email:

2 This expression translates into the current context the Spanish proverb 'muerto el perro, se acabó la rabia' (when the dog is dead, the rabies is gone), the meaning of which is equivalent to the English one, 'dead dogs don't bite'.

References

Agamben, G. (2020), 'L'invenzione di un'epidemia', *Quodlibet*, 26 February. Available online: https://www.quodlibet.it/giorgio-agamben-l-invenzione-di-un-epidemia (accessed 30 October 2020).

Alba Rico, S. (2020), 'Apología del contagio', *Ctxt.es*, 9 March. Available online: https://ctxt.es/es/20200302/Firmas/31282/coronavirus-contagio-apologia-miedo-santiago-alba-rico-covid19-enfermedad.htm (accessed 31 August 2021).

Badiou, A. (2020), 'Sur la situation épidemique', *Cartier Général*. Available online: https://qg.media/2020/03/26/sur-la-situation-epidemique-par-alain-badiou/ (accessed: 30 October 2020).

Deleuze, G. (1990 [1969]), *The Logic of Sense*, trans. M. Lester and C. Stivale, New York: Columbia University Press.
Deleuze, G. (1994 [1968]), *Difference and Repetition*, trans. P. Patton, New York: Columbia University Press.
Deleuze, G. (1995 [1990]), *Negociations 1972–1990*, trans. M. Joughin, New York: Columbia University Press.
Deleuze, G. (1998 [1993]), *Essays Critical and Clinical*, trans. D. W. Smith and M. A. Greco, London: Verso.
Deleuze, G. (2007 [2003]), *Two Regimes of Madness. Texts and Interviews 1975–1995*, trans. A. Hodges and M. Taormina, New York: Semiotext(e).
Deleuze, G. and F. Guattari (1994 [1991]), *What Is Philosophy?*, trans. H. Tomlinson and G. Burchell, New York: Columbia University Press.
Deleuze, G. and F. Guattari (2004 [1980]), *A Thousand Plateaus: Capitalism and Schizophrenia*, trans. B. Massumi, Minneapolis: University of Minnesota Press.
Deleuze, G. and C. Parnet (1987 [1977]), *Dialogues*, trans. H. Tomlinson and B. Habberjam, New York: Columbia University Press.
Descartes, R. (1999), 'Lettre à Hyperaspistes, Agoust 1641', R. Descartes, *Œuvres Philosophiques*. París: Classiques Garnier.
Diéguez, A. (2020), 'Una pandemia sin norte. Los pensadores no levantan cabeza con el coronavirus', *El Confidencial*, 20 March. Available online: https://blogs.elconfidencial.com/cultura/tribuna/2020-03-20/coronavirus-filosofia-pandemia-crisis_2506407/ (accessed 31 August 2021).
Graeber, D. (2020), 'After the Pandemic, We Can't Go Back to Sleep', *Jacobin*, Available online: https://www.jacobinmag.com/2021/03/david-graeber-posthumous-essay-pandemic (accessed 31 August 2021).
Lapoujade, D. (2014), *Deleuze. Les mouvements aberrants*, Paris: Les Éditions du Minuit.
Latour, B. (2019), 'Interview with Bruno Latour', *El País*, 1 April. Available online: https://elpais.com/elpais/2019/03/29/ideas/1553888812_652680.html (accessed 30 October 2020).
Latour, B. (2021), *Où suis-je? Leçons du confinement à l'usage des terrestres*, Paris: La Découverte.
Madrigal, A. (2020), 'The Official Coronavirus Numbers Are Wrong, and Everyone Knows It', *The Atlantic*, 3 March. Available online: https://www.theatlantic.com/technology/archive/2020/03/how-many-americans-really-have-corona virus/607348/ (accessed 29 September 2020).
McIntyre, L. (2018), *Post-Truth*, Cambridge: The MIT Press.
Spanish Ministry of Health (2021), 'Información científica-técnica. Enfermedad por coronavirus, COVID-19'. Available online: https://www.mscbs.gob.es/profesionales/saludPublica/ccayes/alertasActual/nCov/documentos/20210429_GRUPOSPERSONAS.pdf (accessed 1 October 2021).
Nancy, J.-L. (2000 [1995]), *Being Singular Plural*, trans. R. D. Richardson and A. E. O'Byrne, California: Stanford University Press.
Nancy, J.-L. (2020), *Un trop humain virus* [An All Too Human Virus], Paris: Bayard Editions.
Pérez Tapias, J. A. (2020), 'Alternativa: o "común-ismo republicano" o "tanatopolítia"', in D. Tomás Cámara (ed.), *Covidosofía. Reflexiones filosóficas para el mundo postpandemia*, 406–427, Barcelona: Paidós.
Shelton, T. (2020), 'A post-truth pandemic?', *Big Data & Society*, July–December, 1–6.
Žižek, S. (2020), *PANDEMIC! Covid-19 Shakes the World*, New Jersey: Wiley.
Zourabichvili, F. (2012 [1994, 2003]), *Deleuze: A Philosophy of the Event Together with The Vocabulary of Deleuze*, trans. K. Aarons, Edinburgh: Edinburgh University Press.

13

A Cartography of Mutual Aid Groups in Brighton: Ethics of Care and Sustainability

Elizabeth Vasileva

In the UK, the chaotic response of the government to the COVID-19 pandemic coincided with unprecedented levels of grassroots organization and community support. Businesses and organizations, realizing the early threat of the virus, closed before the government had officially ordered lockdown. Individuals and households had already started isolating when Prime Minister Boris Johnson was filmed enthusiastically shaking hands with COVID-19 patients, even before firm guidelines on Covid safety were issued. But what really demonstrated the extent of community action beyond central and local government was the explosion of 'mutual aid' groups across the country through which neighbours, families and businesses shared resources and acted to protect vulnerable, sick and isolating people in their locality. In Brighton, a small-sized city on the south coast of the UK with a population of around 230,000 people, more than 17,000 people joined the mutual aid network, keeping it active for over a year. But what makes such a phenomenon possible?

In this chapter I attempt to map some Deleuze-Guattarian insights onto the mutual aid network in Brighton. Current research on the British mutual aid groups tends to explain the phenomenon through a social representation lens in the form of citizenship (O'Dwyer et al. 2020), community resilience and vulnerability (Matthewman and Huppatz 2020) and identity formation during disasters (Drury 2012). The emergence of the mutual aid groups during the pandemic is likened to other 'disaster responses' where the dominant paradigm for understanding the conditions of emergence comes from social psychology (Fernandes-Jesus et al. 2021). Proponents of this framework understand public behaviour during emergencies as primarily guided by a process of group identity formation. Drury et al. (2019), for instance, identify two main tenets that structure collective behaviour – identities and norms. Their approach is based on the idea that people have a social identity, as well as a personal one. The personal one, perceived as that which makes one unique and 'themselves', is separate from the social one, which comes from our membership in various social groups, such as the group 'women', for instance, or 'students', or 'Deleuzians'. Each social identity carries a certain type of baggage in the form of norms, expectations, values, interests, etc., and not every social identity one has is 'active' at all times, since it is context that makes them relevant (Drury et al. 2019). Theorists advocating for this approach therefore argue that when a disaster or crisis occurs, the 'crowd' develops a shared social identity as 'survivors' of this particular disaster. Social identity, in this sense, is reflexive – one has to see oneself and others as part of it *and* assume that others also view them as part of that group. This new social identity then becomes the driving force for people to help others who are affected by the disaster (Fernandes-Jesus et al. 2021).

While recognizing the importance of collective identity for understanding disaster support and resilience, I would argue that this kind of account is insufficient for understanding the emergence and impact of the mutual aid groups in Brighton. First of all, Drury, for example, claims that 'all those who perceive themselves equally (or "interchangeably") threatened thereby come to categorise themselves as a psychological unit, in relation to that threat' (2012), explaining why people were motived to get involved. However, whilst this might be applicable to situations of immediate danger such as clubhouse members assisting each other to escape a burning building, it struggles to explain a situation where *the whole world* is in danger. The social identity framework implies that everyone now is part of the same identity group as 'covid-survivors' and thus should exhibit solidarity to other members. Second, the social identity approach ignores the particular material and affective factors that contribute to a group's unique formation and gives primacy to the 'disaster' as the (only) generative element of mutual support. For instance, a study of the mutual aid groups in Brighton does not make a single mention of furlough as one of the main elements which enabled participants to volunteer twelve hours a day (Fernandes-Jesus et al. 2021). Third, it analytically isolates the group from everything else that occurs in the same locality, e.g. other groups, the history of the place, the weather, politics, etc. Another study which refers also to Brighton focuses on the use of social media in mutual aid during the pandemic without acknowledging the fact that Brighton already had numerous community social media groups which served a similar function prior to the pandemic and indeed it appears almost all of them remain strong a year and a half into the pandemic (Ntontis et al. 2021). Finally, it examines the group in stasis, rather than in its flows and changes as it responded to the trajectory and development of the virus and the pandemic. Subsequent conclusions, then, are limited and simplify the complexities and uniqueness of the group, as well as failing to fully understand subjectivity-building in relation to community resilience.

To counterpose these kinds of analysis, I propose a new materialist cartography inspired by Deleuze and Guattari's work as a different way of understanding the mutual aid groups in Brighton. A cartography of the present, Rosi Braidotti contests, is a 'theoretically-based and politically-informed account of the present that aims at tracking the production of knowledge and subjectivity, and to expose power both as entrapment and as empowerment' (2019, 33). It is a local and grounded account, selective and partial by necessity and never exhaustive. It understands 'community' as a transversal assemblage incorporating a range of non-human actors, affects and ethics. This framework is particularly pertinent for an Event such as the pandemic, where the non-human actor COVID-19 virus reshaped the world, including socio-political relationships and subjectivities on a micropolitical level. A cartography then helps us see elements of that transformation in the way different actors found themselves reshaped through the mutual aid groups, but also highlight 'how human – but also non-human, more-than-human, and dehumanised – bodies are located within intricate webs of power as *potestas* and potentia' (Gray et al. 2021, 205).

In the children's novel *Peter Pan*, Barrie (1911) describes the following evening activity of Mrs Darling: 'It is the nightly custom of every good mother after her children are asleep to rummage in their minds and put things straight for next morning, repacking into their proper places the many articles that have wandered during the day.' A little bit further on, he describes the mind like a map, one that 'keeps going round all the time'. But it's not just one map, it's actually many different maps on top of each other, all semi-transparent so you can see the one underneath and connected through various lines and roads. Barrie, a contemporary of Freud's, was clearly referring to psychoanalytic attempts to draw maps of the mind. Similarly, schizoanalysis proposes the practice of mapping, while carefully differentiating it from 'tracing'. A tracing means one is trying to fit what is given into a model of what it should be understood as. Tracing is the practice of royal sciences, a theory or a model imposed on the given which abstracts its meaning. Maps, on the other hand, are a feature of rhizomes and will also serve as the basis for a cartography of Brighton's mutual aid groups. The mutual aid network in Brighton was a rhizomatic structure with no centralization or hierarchy which remained extremely active deep into the pandemic. It does not lend itself easily to social psychology tracing without reduction. In Deleuze and Guattari's words:

> The rhizome is altogether different, *a map and not a tracing*. Make a map, not a tracing. The orchid does not reproduce the tracing of the wasp; it forms a map with the wasp, in a rhizome. What distinguishes the map from the tracing is that it is entirely oriented toward an experimentation in contact with the real (1987, 12; emph. in orig.).

A Deleuze-Guattarian cartography is thus best understood as constantly shifting and changing rhizomes, with new connections being formed and various entry and exit points. By using rhizomes as an analytic tool, we can point out contradictions and tension that arises between personal and collective subjectivity. It allows us to see how certain identities are produced through the process, but also how participants adopt them and push against them at the same time. But Deleuze and Guattari's cartography is more than simply a map, a description of various rhizomatic connections. As they say, '*the tracing should always be put back on the map*' (1987, 13; emph. in orig.). In other words, analysis and theory are not separate from what is given; they are not abstractions from the data, but co-exist together and inform each other. As such, this is a continuation of Deleuze's previous rejection of a clear dividing line between theory and practice and Guattari's statement that 'theoretical expressions should function as tool, as machines .... It works or it doesn't work' (Guattari 2000: 22).

So, what would a cartography of the mutual aid network in Brighton tell us that differs from a social identity approach? Is it just a way of noticing different things in research data? Can we move beyond the normative assumptions through which social scientists have come to think of collective identity and community resilience? The challenge for new materialist methodology is to figure out in what ways we are able to say something new and different about the topic. For this chapter I didn't have the scope to do a full cartographic study, but I will nevertheless attempt to sketch some elements which might be considered for one. Being an active mutual aid participant myself (one of the 'reps'), I had privileged access to their functioning and their internal discussions. I have also organized a few follow-up reflections workshops for some of the participants, which has helped build more of a collective narrative of our experiences as organizers. Using Guattari's three ecologies as a starting point, I will experiment with answering the question: What made the mutual aid phenomenon possible in Brighton?

A cartography needs to start with a locality and emphasize the way it is differentiated. Brighton's particularities are contextualized here into each level of Guattari's ecology – environmental, social, mental. It is important to emphasize that the word ecology is specifically selected to show the mutual dependency, interconnections and feedback loops that exist within each register of activity. Thus, the three ecologies of Brighton should not be thought of as separate, but rather as constantly feeding off each other to produce its particular becoming.

The first is the environmental ecology, which focuses on the physical aspects of the environment, although they are not necessarily limited to nature. Our first map then is a geographical map of Brighton. Brighton is a small twin city (with its neighbour Hove) on the south coast of the UK. In this case, size is important as it allows walking access to most places in town for people with sufficient mobility. In the beginning of lockdown, when everyone was advised to not use public transport, walking and cycling were an important factor that enabled the flows of mutual aid. However, Brighton is snuggled in the South Downs, a national reserve known for its hilly make-up. Brighton itself is situated on three hills with its central part in the valley between the three of them. The hills, although a much beloved part of Brighton which contributes to its beauty, also create a barrier for certain bodies, particularly when it comes to delivering heavy bags of shopping from the bottom of a hill to the top.

Brighton's social ecology, on the other hand, includes a very particular mix of liberal, left and radical politics, particularly when it comes to LGBTQ+ organizing. It has often been called 'the gay capital' of the UK and it hosts a number of LGBTQ venues and organizations. It is also the home of various more radical groups, has its own anarchist social centre and a history of working-class organizing. Brighton also hosts a large number of tourists from both the UK and abroad, with the beach serving as a magnet for visitors, partygoers, students and the general Brighton population on a nice summer's day. In keeping with, if not partially responsible for, its liberal/lefty reputation, Brighton claims the only Green Party member of parliament in UK history and has had a Labour- or Green-run Council since 1996. An equally significant element of Brighton's social ecology is its proximity to London. Brighton is about an hour's train journey from the capital, placing it broadly within the commuter belt. This means that a decent volume of the population works in London, receiving London wages (generally higher than anywhere else in the country). Subsequently, this contributes to the relative affluence of central Brighton (near the train station and the commuter motorways), with rent and house prices in the city high in comparison to the regional average. Over time the original town has grown into a small conurbation, connecting to other smaller towns bordering it on the coast, such as Hove, Portslade, Southwick, Woodingdean, etc.[1]

Finally, the particularities of its mental ecology are difficult to express in representational systems of thought like language and perhaps even too difficult for a single individual to conceptualize easily. Guattari himself claims that 'the crucial objective is to grasp the a-signifying points of rupture – the rupture of denotation, connotation and signification – from which a certain number of semiotic chains are put to work in the service of an existential autoreferential effect' (2000, 56). Thus, if I were to try to name some important aspects of the collective psychic ecology of Brighton, I might point to a certain type of subjectivity which celebrates equality, diversity and takes pride in a carefree, relaxed attitude of enjoying life. A commonly seen manifestation of this is dressing in unusual ways, dying one's hair bright or rainbow colours, an incorporation of joyfulness and love of life in one's appearance and lack of shame in relation to bodies. Significantly, Brightonians also value community structures and a DIY ethos of people getting together and changing their environment. All of these constitute forms of rupture of Brighton from much of the rest of conservative East Sussex.

Having applied the three ecologies to the general context of Brighton, we can now use them to inform our analysis of the mutual aid groups and add a second layer to our map. When the pandemic was looming and before the government took any measures, Brighton was one of the first cities in the UK to spring a mutual aid group, which was established in one of the famously bohemian, affluent areas of town. Very quickly, however, these groups spread all over the city. They were rhizomatic in their occurrence and completely self-governed. Anyone could start one and they did not need to ask for permission (although it was advised to make sure there wasn't already one for the area). The material resources required to start one were access to a printer to print out flyers, access to a phone on which people could call to ask for help and the physical ability to distribute the flyers to different households. Often all of this was done collectively by a household or two who wanted to start a mutual aid group. At its peak, Brighton had over eighty networked mutual aid groups with presence on social media. The initial organization consisted of street and/or area 'reps' who met up once a week virtually to report gaps or needs to others, and to work on building community and providing support. Figure 13.2 is a map of the main areas covered by the mutual aid network, or, in other words, a new social ecology of Brighton.

We can now look in a bit more detail at what enabled this phenomenon. Hinting at the limits of the social identity approach, the creation of Brighton's mutual aid network was based on the initial rupture in the collective mental ecology. The Event of COVID-19, hovering over the entire world with its imminent promise of death, transformed the chain of signification of Brighton's mental ecology and snowballed with support from changes in the environmental and social ecology. For instance, the existence of the mutual aid network relied heavily on the ability to not go to work. A large part of the population of the city works in sectors where employees were part of the government furlough scheme through which they were given a proportion of their wages in the first months of the pandemic as material support without having to work (Magrini 2021). This was an extreme example of how a change in the material

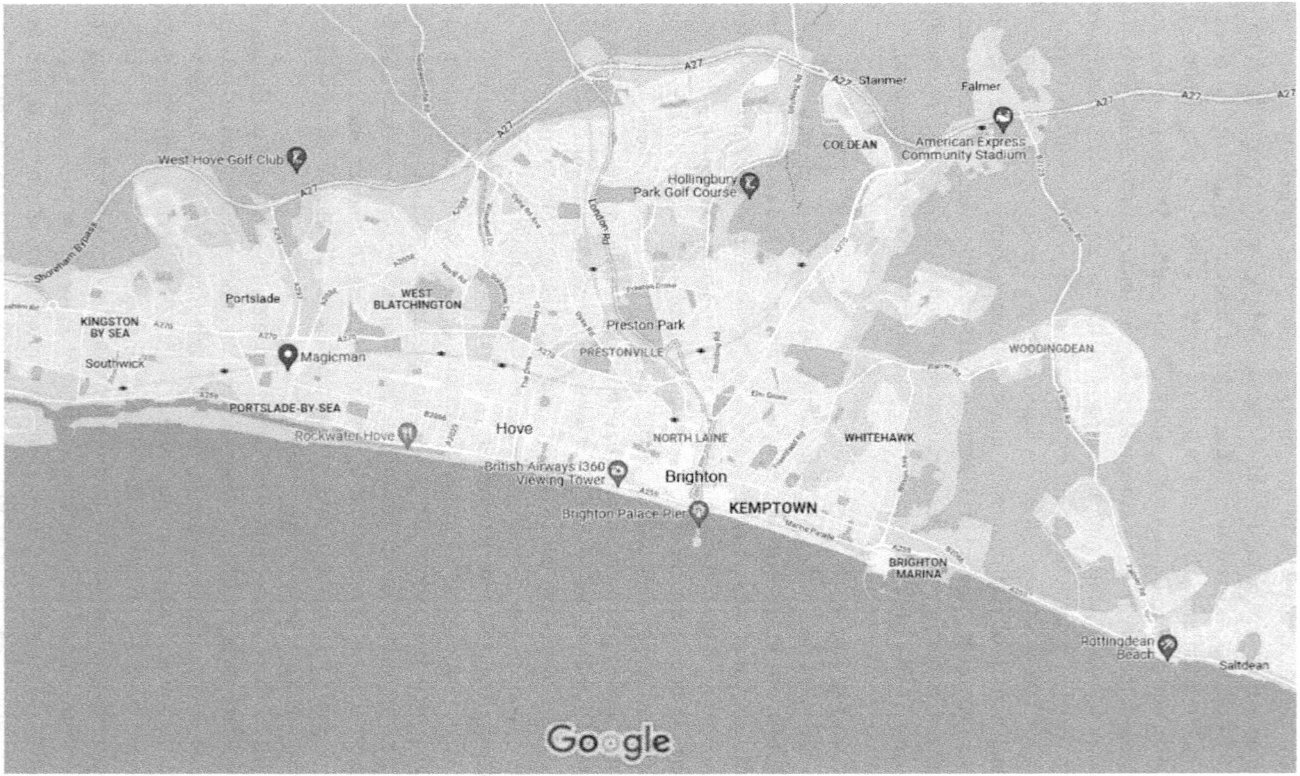

Figure 13.1 A map of Brighton and its conurbation. Map data © 2021. Date accessed: 15 September 2021. https://www.google.com/maps/@50.8362752,-0.1245184,14z

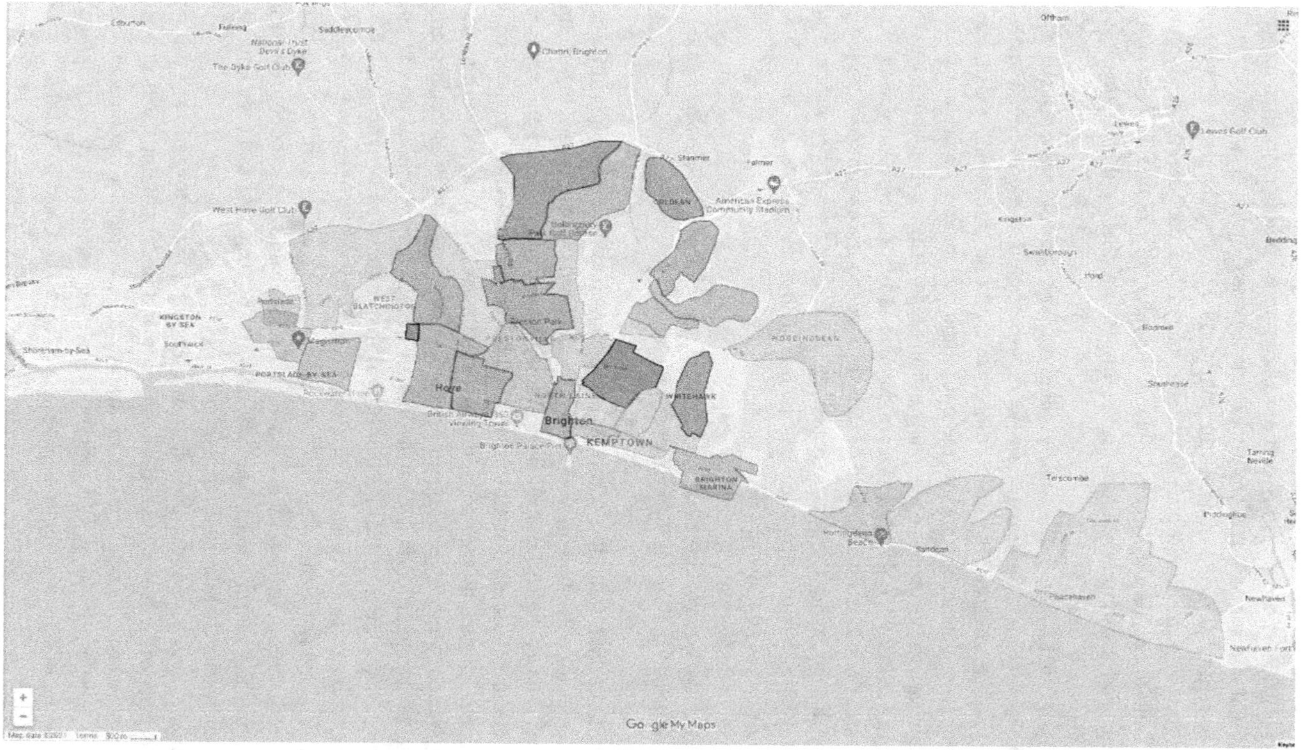

Figure 13.2 A map showing the location of the mutual aid groups in Brighton. Map data © 2021. Date accessed: 15 September 2021. https://www.google.com/maps/@50.8362752,-0.1245184,14z

conditions opened up the possibility for a change in the entire functioning of the city (albeit temporarily). The mutual aid network quickly accumulated a huge number of volunteers (17,500 on social media), some of whom were working more than full-time hours to build and support it. From my experience, most of the reps were either on furlough or retired, as well as most of the volunteers who were involved on a regular basis, and this was something which was often reflected on during meetings. Moreover, with pubs and restaurants being closed, a lot of the volunteers found themselves with a bit of spare cash to support projects in the city, such as the food bank or through driving.

In terms of social ecology, we could perhaps read the pandemic as a 'disaster-actor' within the city. Using a Spinozian framework, for example, Rebecca Solnit analyses how everyday life governed by the joint forces of capitalism and neoliberalism leaves no space for self-determination and the opportunity to increase their ability to act (2009, 2). Disasters, she claims, open a new possibility for trust, responsibility and care by removing certain everyday structures of the state and capitalism. Comparing this to furlough and the sudden withdrawal of structures such as work and commuting, we could see that emptying the space created the possibility for self-organization and community care. For instance, one participant cites the closing down of nurseries as the reason why she got involved:

> My initial idea was to create a 'borrow a granny' network where people who needed to work could just drop off their children with me.

Similarly, the closure of food banks and various mismanagement problems in the care and service sectors left a huge gap which neighbours filled for each other. One example of this was the weekly workshops where mutual aid volunteers would address issues faced by communities often not heard in the everyday mundane experiences of life under neoliberalism. One such workshop centred the voice of a person with no fixed abode who had recently spent some time sleeping on the streets of Brighton. Brighton's rough sleeping population is one of the highest in the country, ranked fifth in 2019 (Ministry of Housing 2020). During this workshop, mutual aid participants heard about the problems faced by rough sleepers in the first months of the pandemic (no access to drinking water after all public taps, cafes and restaurants were shut; no access to health care items due to a combination of closed foodbanks and less opportunity for begging, etc.) and within a week there was an NFA (no fixed address) essentials table established by a local mutual aid rep.

It would be reductive to cite the feeling of 'everyone is in this together' as a primary reason for this collective expression of solidarity and understanding, particularly as participants were increasingly aware of the wealth and comfort discrepancies that meant we were mostly all in different 'this's'. Instead, following Deleuze's Spinozist understanding of power as increasing our capacity to affect and be affected, we can argue that having the space to self-organize produced an increase in collective power (*potenstas*), as *we were able to do things we couldn't do before*. There was a great deal of community-building, joy, connection and solidarity between the participants of the mutual aid network, and a shared feeling that anything was possible. In a Deleuze-

Guattarian framework, perhaps this points to the ways in which having capitalist/neoliberal control abated for a short period of time allowed for a reterritorialization of flows of desire, which resulted in new connections being made, and therefore an increase in collective capacity, collective response-ability and new forms of care that were not possible before. On a micro-political level, volunteers shared endless stories of joy and feeling 'alive' and connected to the world and their locality. One of the reps, for instance, spoke about the reason why she got involved in the mutual aid network rather than the official government structures. Having received medical training (now retired), she was called in by the government to join one of the healthcare sectors where staffing was low. She explains that the existence of the mutual aid network was instrumental in her rejecting the request:

> I decided I could do more in the mutual aid network than I was going to be able to do as a doctor. And I was right because all my friends who signed up to go back were sent to do Track and Trace which failed and they had nothing to do for months whilst we were setting up structures and a huge network and helping lots of people.

This points to the possibility of new social relations being established following the withdrawal of institutionalized actors, but also the efficiency and joyfulness of self-organization.

No cartography can be complete without a mapping of its discursive or meaning-generative elements. The main slogan that informed the mutual aid organizing was 'Solidarity not Charity', clearly visible in its social media and website, together with red and black anarchist symbolism. Although neither the network itself nor its separate groups were politically aligned with a particular ideology (and, in fact, many local groups refused to even discuss 'politics'), its affiliation with anarchism was explicit in its public presence, including an article about anarchist Peter Kropotkin in a newsletter explaining the principles of mutual aid. This was deliberately put in opposition to more traditional or institutionalized charity efforts where financial or material help is distributed to people in need in a top-down fashion. This codifies the relationship between the giver and the receiver to a paternalistic form of entrapment where the need for charitable giving exists for as long as the economic relations remain the same. In other words, people receiving charity are trapped in a system of wealth inequality where they are being denied capacity to affect their conditions.

The rejection of the charity model in the mutual aid network was explicitly built through a common understanding that everyone can contribute to caring for others despite their limitations, affectively increasing the connections we built. Participants could do shopping or cooking for others, but also volunteer to make phone calls with people who were feeling isolated or needed someone to talk to. Some people volunteered to walk others' dogs, pick up medicine, work in a virtual 'office' with others who were finding it hard to be motivated, amongst others. This required a collective reconfiguration of values in the sense of appreciating everyone's efforts equally and not assuming or judging.

This tension between charity and solidarity was perhaps the main productive flow and entrapment for mutual aid participants. People were strongly driven by a desire to avoid the pitfalls of the charity model, whilst at the same time finding it difficult to avoid them entirely. One of the reps, who ended up running a food bank, talked about her efforts to do it differently from other food banks. She mentioned, for instance, deliberately not organizing a system of 'referrals' because they didn't want to judge anyone and wanted to establish trust with the people who used the foodbank. She talked about going through a huge effort to find good-quality food and nice items, such as liaising with local bakeries and restaurants to distribute their leftover food, because she hated the idea that foodbank food just had to be necessities. In fact, this relationship of trust meant that people felt comfortable to tell her, for instance, that they wanted a sourdough bread, because other bread made them bloated, without worrying they would seem ungrateful for what they were given. She explained the success of the food bank in terms of 'giving people choice' through enlisting volunteers to create an app where people could select exactly what food they wanted from the foodbank. She contrasted that with the food parcels which the government sent to people categorized as 'extremely vulnerable' in the beginning of the pandemic. Without taking into account anything about these people, including their financial situation, the government started sending emergency parcels containing basic food items. She explained that often these people would then call her, as a mutual aid rep, and ask her to distribute the food from the parcels to others. They would either receive items they couldn't eat because of their diet, or items they didn't like, or simply things that they already had a lot of.

Similarly, I was coordinating a furniture redistribution hub where people in need could contact me to ask for household items or furniture. I started this group after being made aware that a refugee family of four was sleeping on a mattress on the floor for two months in a mostly unfurnished house at the beginning of the pandemic. To avoid creating a charity relationship whereby the recipients were expected to receive whatever and be grateful, I also ended up asking a volunteer to develop an app so people could choose from the donated furniture and make specific requests, no matter how picky they wanted to be.

A Deleuze-Guattarian framework also exposes how the flows of wealth were often one-sided, from the more affluent inner city to the poorer outskirts, very much in line with a charity model. The next layer of the map shows the approximate locations of where items were coming from and going to. The stars represent families who received furniture, and the lines signify where items came from with a noticeable direction from the affluent centre to the outskirts (Figure 13.3).

The tension within this relationship was productive of a particular kind of subjectivity where one was challenged to think of ways of bypassing the charity model but inherently tied to its limitations. Despite attempts to move beyond and achieve some kind of mutual aid relationship, and despite the collective increase in our capacity to act, the network remained trapped within the limits of minor wealth redistribution. Moreover, the structures established by the network eventually (in some ways) resembled institutionalized efforts. This was particularly evident in questions around safeguarding, for instance, and protecting the identity of people, but also around dogmatic ideological behaviour.

Having reached the limits of this chapter, I can only point to other major actors to be considered in a cartography: the role of technology in setting up and maintaining

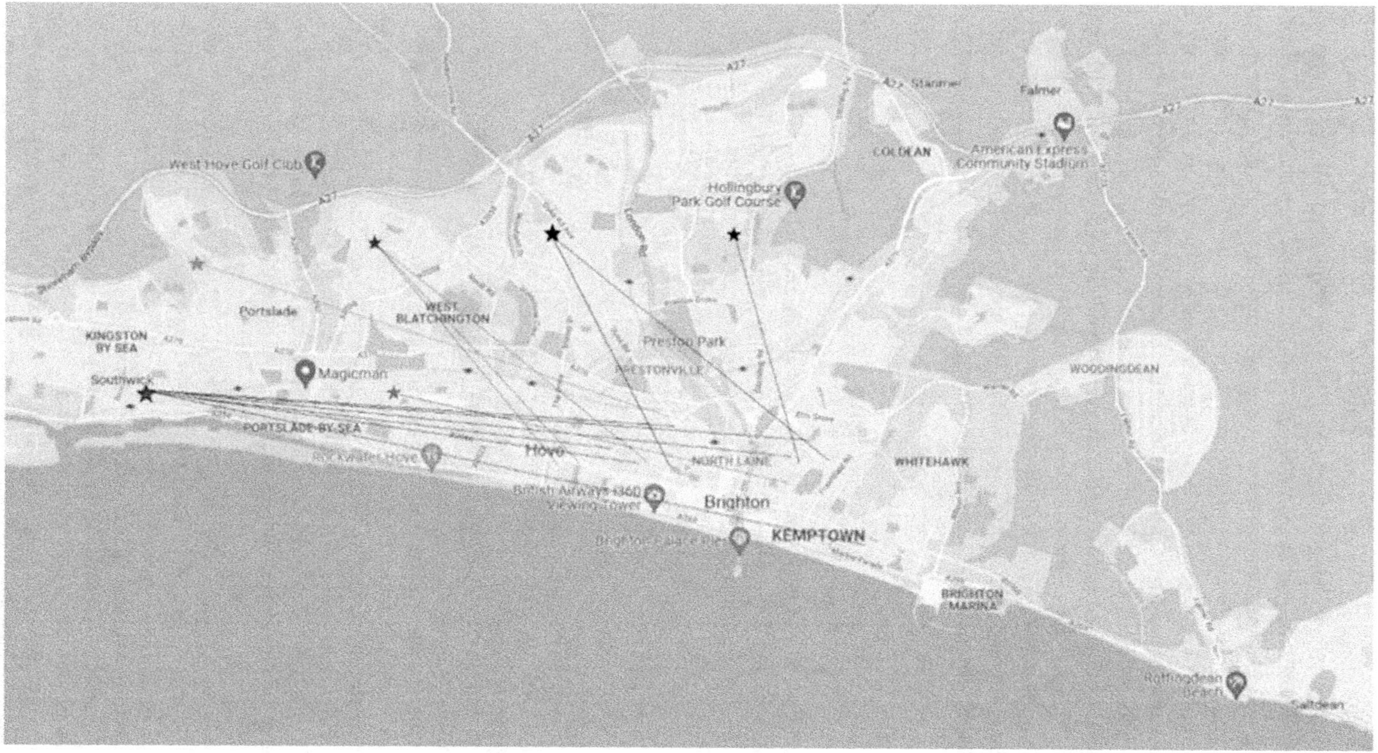

Figure 13.3 A map of Brighton with arrows representing the start and end locations of donated items. Map data © 2021. Date accessed: 15 September 2021. https://www.google.com/maps/@50.8362752,-0.1245184,14z

the network, the trajectory and itinerary of the virus, including the daily deaths and collective psychological affects this caused, the broader context of state regulations and behaviour, the seasonal changes which had an unexpectedly great influence on people's desire to stay at home and coordinate mutual aid activities, the vaccine and ideas of vulnerability, Brexit and the anti-vax movement, among other things. Most importantly, unlike certain social sciences where the 'logic of discursive sets endeavours to completely delimit its objects', the 'logic of intensities, or eco-logic, is concerned only with the movement and intensity of evolutive processes' (Guattari 2000: 44), thus producing an analysis where both the virus and the mutual aid groups are seen as interlocked, feeding off each other and creating endless feedback loops with other elements. This also necessitates understanding the network as a process which was responding to another process. Ultimately these concerns barely approach answers to our initial question, but they offer a significantly more compelling direction than the social identity approaches that are fast becoming a highly cited, go-to narrative.

Note

1 For a more thorough report on Brighton's population and inequalities, please check https://ww3.brighton-hove.gov.uk/sites/brighton-hove.gov.uk/files/downloads/equalities/OCSI_ReducingInequalityReview_phase_1_full_report.pdf

References

Barrie, J. M. (1911/2015), *Peter Pan*, London: Puffin.

Braidotti, R. (2019), 'A Theoretical Framework for the Critical Posthumanities', *Theory, Culture & Society*, *36*(6): 31–61.

Deleuze, G. and Guattari, F. (1987), *A Thousand Plateaus*, Minneapolis: University of Minnesota Press.

Drury, J. (2012), 'Collective Resilience in Mass Emergencies And Disasters: A Social Identity Model' in J. Jetten, C. Haslam, S. A. Haslam and S. Alexander (eds), *The Social Cure: Identity, Health and Well-being*, New York: Psychology Press, 195–215.

Drury, J., Carter, H., Cocking, C., Ntontis, E., Tekin Guven, S. and Amlot, R. (2019), 'Facilitating Collective Psychosocial Resilience in the Public in Emergencies: Twelve Recommendations Based on the Social Identity Approach', *Frontiers in Public Health* 7 (1): 141.

Fernandes-Jesus, M., Mao, G., Ntontis, E., Cocking, C. McTague, M., Schwarz, A., Semlyen, J. and Drury, J. (2021), 'More than a COVID-19 Response: Sustaining Mutual Aid Groups During and Beyond the Pandemic', *SocArXiv*, 29 May. Available online: https://osf.io/preprints/socarxiv/p5sfd/ (accessed 14 October 2021).

Gray, C., Carstens, D., Geerts, E. and Eloff, A. (2021), 'Deleuzoguattarian Thought, the New Materialism, and (Be)wild(erring) Pedagogies: A Conversation between Chatelle Gray, Delphi Carstens, Evelien Geerts, and Aragorn Eloff', *Matter: Journal of New Materialist Research* 2(1): 200–223.

Guattari, F. (2000), *The Three Ecologies*, London: Athlone Press.

Magrini, E. (2021), 'Which Jobs Are Currently Most Reliant on the Coronavirus Job Retention Scheme in the Largest Cities and Towns?', *Centre for Cities*, 30 March. Available online: https://www.centreforcities.org/blog/which-jobs-are-currently-most-reliant-on-the-coronavirus-job-retention-scheme-in-the-largest-cities-and-towns/ (accessed 14 October 2021).

Matthewman, S. and Huppatz, K. (2020), 'A Sociology of Covid-19', *Journal of Sociology*, 56(4): 675–683.

Ministry of Housing (2020), 'Rough Sleeping Snapshot in England: Autumn 2019', *Official Statistics*. 27 February. Available online: https://www.gov.uk/government/statistics/rough-sleeping-snapshot-in-england-autumn-2019/rough-sleeping-snapshot-in-england-autumn-2019 (accessed 14 October 2021).

Ntontis, E., Fernandes-Jesus, M., Mao, G., Dines, T., Kane, J., Karakaya, J., Rotem Perach, R., Cocking, C., McTague, M., Schwarz, A., Semlyen, J. and Drury, J. (2021), 'Tracking the Contours and Nature of Social Support in Facebook Mutual Aid Groups During the COVID-19 Pandemic', *PsyArXiv*, 8 October. Available online: https://psyarxiv.com/vedn3/download/?format=pdf (accessed 14 October 2021).

O'Dwyer, E., Silva-Souza, L., and Beascoech-Segui, N. (2020), 'Rehearsing Post-covid-19 Citizenship: Social Representations and Social Practices in UK Mutual Aid Groups.' *PsyArXiv*, 10 December. Available online: https://psyarxiv.com/v84mr/ (accessed 14 October 2021).

Solnit, R. (2009), *A Paradise Built in Hell: The Extraordinary Communities that Arise in Disaster*, New York: Penguin Books.

Index

Note: References followed by "n" refer to endnotes.

www.ingramcontent.com/pod-product-compliance
Lightning Source LLC
Chambersburg PA
CBHW052112300426
44116CB00010B/1631
9781350277397